TABLE OF CONTENTS

PAGES

LIST OF FIGURES AND TABLES

FOREWORD

I first met Professor Lawrence A. Adeokun in the academic context at the Rockefeller Foundation South-South Retreat in Bellagio, Italy in 1989. He was one of two African social scientists the Foundation invited to give advice on how best to proceed with some aspects of the South-South Initiative. He was impressive. He was at the peak of his career both as a staff of Obafemi Awolowo University (OAU), Ile-Ife and as an international scholar then serving as the first Senior Representative for Anglophone Sub-Saharan Africa at the Population Council Office in Nairobi, Kenya.

When he retired from OAU and returned to Nigeria after his stay at the Institute of Statistics and Applied Economics (ISAE), Makerere University, Kampala, Uganda where he was a Visiting Professor, ARFH approached him to join the organisation as Director of the Evaluation and Operations Research (E&OR) Unit. Our expectation was that he would add value to the organisation and also provide leadership to the group of young talented staff in the Unit, some of whom were his former students. He did not disappoint us.

His presence in ARFH facilitated the approval of some competitive as well as invited proposals virtually from the day he joined the organisation. Surprisingly, his work ethics was not that of an acknowledged scholar but that of an energetic and committed intellectual. Some of his younger colleagues were had put keeping up with his physical and intellectual energy. But because of his disposition he was able to build a team around him that consistently attained project objectives and had evidence to show for it. His emphasis was on the quality of outputs not on volume. Major publications and international abstracts were completed during his tenure which ended on February 1, 2010 at the age of 71.

On the academic leadership front, it is significant that most of the staff who worked with him in the E&OR Unit now hold important positions in International NGOs. In addition, he assisted in the supervision of the Ph.D. and Master's theses of some members of staff of ARFH. But much more was to come. In November 2010 at the First National Family Planning Conference in Abuja, ARFH arranged for the launching and distribution of his book on Sociocultural Aspects of Family Planning and HIV/AIDS in Nigeria with support from the United Nations Population Fund (UNFPA) Office in Nigeria.

I was not aware that more was to come still. Consequently it was with great pleasure that I accepted to write the Foreword to this publication titled Changing Behaviour in an Epidemic in the Era of HIV/AIDS and Ebola Virus Disease. What Part I of the book does is to present the core of the theoretical framework within which Professor Adeokun executed all the projects for which he was Principal Investigator during his 12 years at ARFH. At every project meeting and feedback he explained the purpose of the framework with conviction and enthusiasm. Approaches to behaviour change communication tended to focus on some elements of the process of change and not on others. The characteristics of a largely traditional and unsophisticated population make some of the assumptions of classic Western models and frameworks not fully applicable to the Nigerian setting. This was what his 4-stage framework of behaviour change tackled on the HIV prevention projects.

In Part II he has shown how events on five major sub-projects for which the AIDS Prevention Initiative in Nigeria (APIN) and the World AIDS Foundation, Paris, France provided substantial and sustained support allowed him and his project team to show the proof of concept of his framework and validate and develop it into a locally relevant tool of behaviour change. With the Ebola virus outbreak he added a final chapter which reviews the possibilities of the same framework for behaviour change serving the purpose of such a fast moving event as the Ebola Virus Disease (EVD) outbreak. He ends by suggesting the application to some of the intractable problems of sexual and reproductive health. It makes interesting discussion.

Anyone reading the book will appreciate the clarity of ideas and of execution that makes his 4-stage framework worthy of consideration in the Public Health and Health Education curriculum of our Colleges of Medicine. We wish him God's blessings and guidance in his future activities which may well include further surprises from a demographer who turns 76 next January. Great indeed is God's faithfulness.

Professsor O.A. Ladipo, FRCOG, OON
President/CEO
Association for Reproductive and Family Health (ARFH)
Plot 815A, Army Officers' Mess Road
Near Ikolaba Grammar School
Agodi G.R.A., Ikolaba, Ibadan
P.O. Box 30259. Secretariat
Ibadan, Oyo State Nigeria

ACKNOWLEDGEMENT

PROJECT FUNDING
The funding for the projects discussed in chapters 5 to 9 of this book are "Promoting Dual Protection Practices in Nigeria" implemented by the Association for Reproductive and Family Health (ARFH) between 1998 and 2000 with funding from the World's AIDS Foundation, Paris; and "The involvement of Male partners of Family Planning clients in Dual Protection promotion" implemented from 2000 to 2001 with support from HORIZONS.

"The AIDS Prevention Initiatives in Oyo State, Nigeria" was implemented by ARFH from 2000 to 2002 with support from AIDS Prevention Initiative in Nigeria (APIN). "The Promotion of HIV Prevention among Most at Risk Populations (MARPS)" sub-projects were implemented by ARFH from 2000 to 2003 also with support from AIDS Prevention Initiative in Nigeria (APIN). And the "HIV Surveillance in four Ogbomosho and Ibadan Markets" was implemented by ARFH and the Department of Virology, College of Medicine, University College Hospital, Ibadan from 2003 to 2005 with support from APIN and with Professor David Olaleye as co-investigator. Thereafter, APIN also supported the operations of two stand alone Voluntary Counselling and Testing clinics in Ibadan and Ogbomosho from 2005 to 2010.

The substantial and sustained support from the APIN in the course of 10 years from 2000 to 2010 was critical to the conceptualization of the 4-stage Framework for Behaviour Change and the progress from Proof of Concept to the validation and evaluation of Framework for Behaviour Change. The conceptualization processes are described in Part I of this book and the application of the HIV prevention sub-projects and activities form the background to Part II. Without this support the effectiveness of the framework would have been pure speculation.

Project Leadership
Professor O.A. Ladipo was the Project Director; Chief Grace E. Delano was the Deputy Director and Professor L. A. Adeokun was the Principal Investigator for all the projects and co Investigator with Professor David Olaleye of the Department of Virology, UCH, Ibadan on the HIV Surveillance project in Ibadan and Ogbomoso.

Project Teams
On the "Dual Protection project" were Grace Ebun Delano, Lawrence Adeokun, Eugene Weiss (Former Member Board of Trustees), Joanne E. Mantell (then research scientist at the HIV Center for Clinical & Behavioral Studies, New York State Psychiatric Institute, Columbia University, New York, and senior research associate at the New York Academy of Medicine, New York.), Ellen Weiss (then research utilization director for the Horizons Programme and a staff member of the International Center for Research on Women, Washington, DC.) and the following former staff of the Association for

Reproductive and Family Health, Ibadan, Nigeria: Stella Akinso, Temple Jagha, Jumoke Olatoregun, Dora Udo.

On other APIN-ARFH Projects were the following former and current staff of ARFH: Mary Iretioluwa Sutton, Kayode Akinpelu, Oluwatoyin Sadiq, Frank Oransanye, Niyi Olaleye, Labake Oguntokun, Solomon Ojeaga, Bidemi Edu, Funmilayo Adediji, Kemi Eludipo, Rashidat Alonge, Kunle Agunbiade, and others.
APIN-ARFH Project Markets

The eight project markets were Owode Market, Anajere Market, Bola Ige Market, Gate Market, Oje market, and Mokola Market all in Ibadan and Aaradaa Market, Ojatuntun Market, and Oja Oba all in Ogbomoso, Oyo State.

Without the cordial working relationships and atmosphere created by these individuals and the population of the Project Markets, the operations research activities of the type described in this book would have been impossible. My gratitude goes to the following people who with their substantive suggestions and careful reading of drafts saved me from obvious pitfalls: Professor Ademola J. Ajuwon, Mrs. Olayimika Adebola and Mrs. O. Oduola.
Above all, to Dr. Prosper Okonkwo, CEO, APIN, Abuja, Nigeria, a reliable friend and support in times of need, I express my profound appreciation.

ACRONYMS

AIDS	Acquired Immunodeficiency Syndrome
AGPMPN	Association of General Private Medical Practitioners of Nigeria
APIN	AIDS Prevention Initiative in Nigeria
APIIOS	AIDS Prevention Initiative in Oyo State
ARFH	Association for Reproductive and Family Health
ARPS	At Risk Populations
ARV	Anti-retroviral
BCC	Behaviour Change Communication
BCT	Behaviour Change Theories
CBD	Community Based Distribution
CCTV	Closed Circuit Television
CDC	Center for Disease Control and Prevention
CHEW	Community Health Extension Worker
CP	Change Process
CSW	Commercial Sex Workers
DP	Dual Protection
ELPE	Extended Life Planning Education
EVD	Ebola Virus Disease
FC	Female Condom
FCMC	First Consultants Medical Centre
FGC	Female Genital Cutting
FIIP	Female Initiated Protection Paradigm
FP	Family Planning
HBM	Health Belief Model
HIV	Human Immunodeficiency virus
IDUs	Intravenous drug users
IEC	Information Education and Communication
IUCD	Intra Uterine Contraceptive Device
LGA	Local Government Authority
MARPS	Most at Risk Population
MIG	Male Involvement Group
MIS	Management Information System
MSM	Men having Sex with Men
NGO	Non Governmental Organisation
NIH	National Institute of Health
OC	Organisation Control
PE	Peer Educator
PEPFAR	President's Emergency Plan for AIDS Relief
PHC	Primary Health Centre
PLWHA	Persons Living with HIV and AIDS
KAP	Knowledge, Attitude and Practice

SL/CT	Social Learning/Cognitive Theory
SRH	Sexual and Reproductive Health
STDs	Sexually Transmitted Diseases
STIs	Sexually Transmitted Infections
TB	Tuberculosis
TPA	Theory of Planned Action
TPB	Theory of Planned Behaviour
TRA	Theory of Reasoned Action
UCH	University College Hospital
UNAIDS	Joint United Nations Programme on HIV and AIDS
USA	United States of America
VCT	Voluntary Counselling and Testing
WAF	World's AIDS Foundation
WHO	World Health Organisation

INTRODUCTION

I n spite of the title of this book, it is not about HIV and AIDS. It is about the difficult task of making people change their behaviour even when there is overwhelming evidence that what they do in their sexual life and other social practices is directly linked to the risk of being infected and of either surviving the infection or dying from it. In over three decades since the first identification of the HIV much is now known about the possible source of the virus, its transmission in human populations, the prevention of transmission and the detection, treatment, management and care of the infected individual. Out of this body of knowledge has emerged the realization that although the infection can be deadly, and left undetected and unmanaged in all probability leads to a devastating AIDS and eventual death, it is preventable, treatable and survivable provided the general population and the infected individuals make the logical and necessary changes which are now generally well known.

In simple terms the state of scientific knowledge about these issues can be codified. On the biomedical aspects these are the basic issues to be taken into consideration:

1. HIV is a retrovirus but not the only one that affects human population.
2. The difficulty of determining the incubation period for HIV is that it can be defined as either the time between exposure to the virus and the first appearance of symptoms or the period between exposure to HIV and progression to full-blown Acquired Immunodeficiency Syndrome (AIDS). Only in rare cases can the time of exposure to the virus be well defined except for those who had unique circumstances of exposure such as work place pin prick, visit to dental or similar appointments which result in an exposure, blood transfusion or equally unique sexual encounter which facilitates the timing of exposure. Similarly, without awareness of the exposure to the virus, the appearance of symptoms may not be linked with the fact of infection. Consequently, the incubation period is an estimate based on the history of those who have clear idea of time of exposure and who, because they go for HIV test, have the appearance of symptoms recognised for what it is.
3. On average, the HIV incubation period in adults is estimated at between one and six months depending on the genetic makeup, the prompt diagnosis, care and treatment, adherence of the individual to treatment and prevention and prompt response to drug resistance among other factors.
4. Various illnesses, called opportunistic infections, can manifest as a result of the decline in immune capacity and inadequately treated or not treated at all produce further decline in the immune system, ending with the protracted incapacitation of the human host and eventual death.
5. The fatality from untreated infection varies, depending on the immune levels and life styles of the individual and depending on the baseline level of immune

system at the time of infection. Consequently, the infection can be social group selective.

6. But detected early and appropriate treatment commenced on time, the infection can be survived and the infected person can live a normal life and die of old age or non-HIV related disease.

7. Because of the transmissibility of infection from mothers to their infants, early detection of the HIV status of the pregnant woman can allow the prevention of that vertical transmission and the survival of the mother.

The main social behavioural features of HIV and AIDS that emerged over the years are:

1. The majority of infections are the result of sexual transmission, irrespective of the orientation of that sexual activity which may be homo or heterosexual in nature.

2. Less than five in a hundred infections can be the result of other avenues of exchanging infected body fluids such as through transmission of infected blood, injection needle prick in the health care setting, exchange of needles among intravenous drug users and transmission in skin piercing practices such as circumcision and female genital cutting with infected cutting instruments.

3. The strategy for prevention varies with the different sources of infection and, therefore, the most dominant issue in HIV prevention is the need for sexual behaviour change and adoption of other behaviour and practices which can assist prevention or assure survival of infection.

4. Since the path of sexual transmission is the exchange of body fluids during unprotected sexual intercourse, that is, without the use of a barrier that prevents the exchange, the most frequently advocated behaviour change for prevention of sexual transmission is the abstinence from sexual intercourse or the use of condoms (male or female condom) or other barrier methods such as foams, gel or suppositories with virucidal agents.

5. Although not every sexual act between an HIV infected individual and an uninfected partner produces transmission, the probability of infection and the consequences of infection make prophylactic sexual practices advisable in every sexual act.

6. Away from sexual transmission, the adoption of safety measures in skin piercing activities in both health care system and in traditional practices also require a change of behaviour away from what was the usual practice to what is the safe practice.

During the course of infection a number of additional biomedical and social guidelines are provided to slow the rate of replication of the virus, reinforce the immune status and further reduce the production of new infections by those who are infected. A number of such guidelines are that:

a. The infected individual keeps all mandatory appointments at the prescribed health facility from the time of detection of HIV status essentially for the rest of their life, given the state of knowledge about the management of the disease.
b. Appropriate arrangements be made by the health facility to monitor the progress of treatment and make prompt detection and appropriate response to drug resistance.
c. The treatment of opportunistic infections in HIV infected individuals and the provision of care and support are aimed at achieving the desired health outcomes.

In effect, this rigorous adherence to health care conditions is not exactly second nature to people who are not used to leading a regimented life. The dilemma for HIV/AIDS prevention, management care is that alteration of "routine practices", "habits" or "behaviour" does not come easy and for many people it is irritating and unachievable. The purpose of this book is twofold: In the first part of the book, we explore in Chapter 1 the distinction between outbreaks and epidemic. Chapter 2 discusses what habits are. Then in Chapter 3 follows the review of existing Western theories and models of behaviour change. One outcome of the review is the revelation of the extent to which the models are not appropriate for application in non-Western traditional populations for which they were not primarily designed. The other outcome was the felt need for an intuitive staged behaviour change that is more suitable for non-Western population. In Chapter 4, an elaboration of the 4-stage intuitive model of behaviour change that is tailored to the world view of the Yoruba of southwest Nigeria is presented. The materials and methods needed for the implementation of the different stages are also discussed in this chapter.

In Part I the focus is on the theoretical origins and links between the 4-Stage Intuitive model and the group of Health Belief Model (HBM) and theories. In contrast, Part II is concerned with how the 4-stage model evolved from the practical application and adaptation of the theories to research projects on HIV prevention among target population groups. This process is in the research traditional cycle of starting with theory in the implementation of interventions and discovering that, most often, the theory does not fit the situation perfectly, requiring that there be gathering of new information with which to modify the theory. The outcome is to make the theory more robust in subsequent application.

Part II of the book is made up of the evolution, application and evaluation of the 4-stage framework on projects of HIV prevention through effecting behaviour change in three major towns in southwest Nigeria, namely, Lagos, Ibadan and Ogbomoso. In Chapters 6 to 9, the sequence of events making up the behaviour change communication programme in five different social platforms in Ibadan using the intuitive model is presented. The impact of the target population on the adjustment of the models over time is also presented to reveal the robustness of the 4-stage framework. Attention is paid to the prescribed social norms of interaction at each platform so that communication can be effective and reception assured as preconditions to progressing along the stages of behaviour change.

In Chapter 5 the focus is on the project titled Promoting Dual Protection in six Ibadan Family Planning Clinics. Stated briefly, dual protection (DP), is the concept of adopting the use of barrier methods of contraception as a means of solving the two associated outcomes of being sexually active, namely, getting pregnant when the woman does not want to get pregnant and getting a sexually transmitted infection including HIV/AIDS at the same time. Two barrier contraceptive methods were promoted on the project. These were the familiar male condom and the comparatively new female condom which was developed only in the course of the last decade and a half of the 20th century and with limited circulation and evaluation of its acceptability (Bounds W, et.al., 1988; Farr, G, et.al., 1994; Trussell, 1998). In contrast the male condom has been around in one form or another for centuries (Cichocki M., 2006; Adeokun, 2009).

Why is condom programming essential for HIV prevention?

In the fight against the continuing spread of HIV/AIDS, Nigeria has made major strides in the treatment of HIV infection with anti-retroviral drugs (ARVs) and in significantly improving the quality of life of people living with the virus. But such treatment and benefits are currently only available for 40% of those with HIV/AIDS. For the majority, the ARV services remain inaccessible (FMOH, 2010). It is also apparent that the prospects of a preventive vaccine or cure for HIV/AIDS are far in the future.

On the prevention side, since the vast majority of adults and young people acquire HIV/AIDS through unprotected sexual intercourse, one of the most accessible options is the reduction of exchange of bodily fluids between sexual partners. For this, the main prevention strategy is based on encouraging safer sexual behaviour including condom use.

The risk of HIV infection is 2 to 9 times greater when other sexually transmitted infections (STIs) are present. Consistent and correct use of condoms, both male and female, is a proven highly effective means of protection from HIV infection, most other STIs, and unintended pregnancy. There is sufficient evidence to demonstrate that consistent and correct condom use reduces the risk of HIV infection considerably, ranging from 60% to 96%. International consensus documents affirm prevention as the mainstay of any response to the HIV epidemic and condoms as an essential part of prevention programming (UNFPA, 2002).

Although people understand the logic behind the recommendation of the use of barrier methods to stop the sexual spread of the HIV, there are various challenges facing the popularisation of such methods, especially the male and female condoms. These include the following:

Health service provider attitudes can influence potential condom users

Many providers view condoms only for their role as contraceptives, downplaying or ignoring their infection prevention properties. Often, when faced with recommending contraceptive choices, providers choose methods that are less user-dependent at the time of sexual relations, such as injectables or oral contraceptive pills. Some providers are openly uncomfortable discussing condoms, will not discuss condoms, or are biased against unmarried youth obtaining condoms. Peer Counsellors are often better able to relate to the potential condom user, facilitating discussions.

Myths, misperceptions and fears hinder access to and use of condoms.

The readiness to use condoms is influenced by personal attitudes that are partly shaped by the socio-cultural environment. Condoms are sometimes associated with promiscuity, feared to be ineffective against HIV, or simply disliked. Ignorance of HIV or perceived low risk of becoming infected also contributes to the reticence to use condoms. Myths such as 'condoms are HIV-contaminated' can influence perceptions of entire communities. Providing correct information and knowledge is important, though often insufficient to alter behaviour which requires finding what motivates people to use condoms consistently and correctly, and programming to stimulate and sustain this incentive.

Inadequate promotion of condoms

Encouraging the use of condoms as dual protection requires that they be promoted for their contraceptive effect as well as for their STI prevention. Studies indicate that when promoted as a means of dual protection, interest in condom use increases. Counsellors should inform clients of the risks of STIs/HIV, potential condom failures and chances of unwanted pregnancy, and back-up such as emergency contraception. Unfortunately, competing priorities, especially at the country level, often leave few resources – financial or human - available for condom programming.

Two features of the DP project are directly related to these difficulties facing the adoption of family planning in general and of barrier methods in particular. First, the decision to work with women in family planning clinics was based on the recognition that this was an easier approach than starting the promotion in the general population. Women attending family planning clinics, for whatever reason, have moved along the chain of events that leads to changing sexual and reproductive behaviour. They have recognised in their own lives, with a little help from family planning promotion, that either the number of children or the timing of births created difficulties in their lives; they also were informed about the ability of family planning clinics to help them; they had access to such clinics and took advantage of the clinics by seeking information and services from the clinics.

Although these steps taken by the women appear like a crude approximation of the 4-stage model, in reality, as survey evidence over the years show, there were various stumbling blocks along the way for such women (Bulatao 1998). First is the impact of prevailing cultural and social norms among Nigerians in which most women do not recognise that their family size poses any problem. There is in fact a conscious effort to have as many children as possible and the only occasion for alarm is when a woman fails to have children. In some circumstances, the family size is actually regarded as a blessing (Adeokun, 1987). Another problem identified was lack of knowledge about the use of contraception and how it is used and where services are available. A quarter of women whose desire for contraception was not met cited this problem.

Second is the concern about the health effects of contraception, cited by one-fifth of the respondents in the study for their unmet needs for contraception. Third is that limited supplies and out of stock syndrome relating to contraceptives often led to unmet needs of women who have access to clinics.

These cultural and familial barriers to family planning can influence a woman's decision to use contraception. Husband may disapprove because he wants more children or is concerned about health effects. He may also base his objection purely on a selfish motive of avoiding the constraints on his sexual life imposed by the need for contraception and prevention of infection. His decision may, in effect, be uninformed. Finally, the family planning programmes often face challenges of providing effective services such as the high rate at which some clients discontinue use of contraception they have been provided. Such discontinuation may also be the outcome of the limitations of the counselling they were given by providers in the first place or the poor or lack of suitable alternative contraceptives. Discontinuation may also be based on religious or cultural grounds or objections from the male partner.

However, when women for any reason find that there are difficulties in their lives arising from the number of children they have or in the timing of pregnancies, they may be willing to do something about those difficulties. But unfortunately, they may have no information as to what to do because of their rural residence or because of their illiteracy. These characteristics prevent them from accessing some family planning promotional materials which are placed in the print or electronic media. The fact of illiteracy may reduce comprehension of the promotional messages. This may create fear of family planning options on the basis of hearsay, distortion of meaning of message and the preclusion of a truly informed consent (Adeokun, 2009).

Consequently, going to the family planning clinic does not mean ac}ceptance of a method. Acceptance of a method does not mean the acceptance of the most reliable method as less than 2% of Nigerian women who are using any method of family planning accept the hormonal and other long lasting methods (NDHS, 2010 etc.). A further complication arises with use of barrier methods which the project focussed on as the most effective against the transmission of HIV. These barrier methods, and in particular the female condom, requires the concurrence of the sexual partner as it is difficult to understand how a woman can use the female condom in its current forms without the partner noticing its presence. This requirement of seeking the concurrence of the sexual partner in the use of the female condom turned out, on the project, to be a major problem even for women who were enthusiastic about the method. The difficulty of convincing males to use the male condom as a prophylactic devise to prevention HIV and other infections remained a major obstacle to female use as it had been over the years.

In short, there were substantial obstacles that the project needed to overcome if the objective of improved use of barrier methods in all sexual encounters is to be achieved. The strategy adopted was the Female Initiated Protection Paradigm (FIPP) (Adeokun, et al., 2002) which required that the female clients will go through this behaviour change cycle so as to be able to take on the challenge of sharing their conviction about the adoption of female condoms with their sexual partners.

It was against the background of the difficulties of FP promotion that the projects described in the following four chapters reveal how the application of the 4-stage framework was put to use to overcome the various challenges. The projects were "Promoting Dual Protection Practices in Nigeria" implemented by the Association for Reproductive and Family Health (ARFH) between 1998 and 2000 with funding from the World's AIDS Foundation, Paris; "The involvement of male partners of FP clients in DP promotion" implemented from 2000 to 2001 with support from HORIZONS; and the ARPS projects implemented from 2000 to 2003 and the follow up "HIV Surveillance in four Ogbomoso and Ibadan Markets" from 2003 to 2005 both with support from the AIDS Prevention Initiative in Nigeria (APIN). In response to the favourable outcomes of these projects and in particular, the last two, APIN supported the operations of two stand alone VCT clinics and an integrated VCT services in Ibadan and Ogbomoso from 2005 to 2010.

These project summaries demonstrate how the 4-stage framework evolved and was consolidated into the behaviour changing tool which it became. In the last but one chapter 9, the impact of the 4-stage framework on the outcomes of the various projects is evaluated in terms of the performances of the operations of three VCT clinics in Ogbomoso and Ibadan from 2005 to 2010 and the integrated VCT clinic based in the ARFH Main clinic which is still in service after the closure of the project linked services in the two other clinics.

In Chapter 9 the operations of two stand alone VCT clinics in Ogbomoso and Ibadan under one of the HIV prevention projects and an integrated VCT clinic operated within ARFH clinic are evaluated so as to show the extent to which the decision to take the HIV test is a logical outcome of the process of staging behaviour change within the 4-stage framework. And the recommendations regarding the potential public health applications of the framework are presented.

This was to have been the full scope of the book until the advent of the Ebola Virus Disease in Nigeria raised the intellectual issue of the relevance of the 4-stage framework to an outbreak which could potentially transmute into an epidemic. The sequence of events in three months between the arrival of the Patient Zero on July 20, 2014 and his death on July 25 and the final declaration by the World Health Organisation that Nigeria was Ebola free on October 20, 2014 form the bulk of the final Chapter 10.

The circumstances in which behaviour change communication and practices conflict with the model are identified and the needed changes to those practices recommended. The need for appropriate sequencing of messages is the major issue discussed in this context. The worrying ethical issues raised by the urgency of responses to a deadly contagion are also discussed. Finally the potential to extend the application of the framework to the management of other health problems is suggested.

PART I

DEVELOPMENT OF THE 4-STAGE INTUITIVE FRAMEWORK

CHAPTER 1
OUTBREAKS AND EPIDEMICS

The starting point for a discussion of behaviour change as a strategy for health improvement is the distinction between an isolated health/disease event and a true epidemic. Outbreaks of diseases with or without an accompanying fatality are such events. They remain outbreaks if they are not sustained over a long period of time. When such outbreaks occur, the health system goes into three sequences of interventions which are fairly predictable. First is the study of the cases, patterns and histology of the disease. Second is the accumulation of the findings from the studies so that analysis can be made as to the possible prevention, diagnoses, treatment and management of cases and the potential for the control of further spread of the disease and the prevention of future outbreaks. The final stage is an assessment of the extent to which these earlier steps have succeeded in bringing the outbreak under control such that the disease is, for the time being, no longer a public health threat. However vigilance, including some degree of behaviour modification and change may be needed to prevent the reoccurrence of the outbreak.

There are occasions, however, when what is thought to be an outbreak does not respond to these stages of public health response. The causative agent responsible for the outbreak may be unknown. It may take time to find out and meanwhile the outbreak spreads and crosses local and national barriers. And by the time the local and international effort to establish the appropriate responses for the prevention, diagnosis, treatment and management and put in place the necessary health system requirements the spread of the disease has gone beyond the original area of outbreak. In such circumstances, the original outbreak transforms into a global epidemic.

It is worth looking at this system of reclassification from an international perspective and especially through the prism of the World Health Organisation that has the mandate for such determination of the status of outbreaks. For now, we could use the cases of two diseases to make vital systems distinction between outbreak and epidemic. The two diseases are Ebola and HIV/AIDS, both with strong association with the continent of Africa. In the past decade (2000 to 2010) the Democratic Republic of Congo experienced more than 5 outbreaks of Ebola fever each lasting between 2 and 6 months (CDC, 2010) but generating a frenetic response from the local and international health community. Because of the self limiting nature of the outbreaks which occurred in remote communities of the Congo, Ebola fever does not attain the status of an epidemic. In contrast, because of the global distribution of HIV infection and AIDS, its rapid spread and slow progress towards its control and management, HIV is classified not only as an epidemic but a "pandemic".

There are similarities and differences between HIV and Ebola Hemorrhagic Fever (EHF). Both are viral infections; both are deadly. The fatality rate of recorded EHF in the first decade of the 21st century is between 50% and 88%. But whilst the outbreak and conclusion of EHF is usually a matter of months, the long gestation of HIV and variable progression to AIDS and death means that HIV is a slowly evolving epidemic whilst the EHF episodes are outbreaks. Consequently, the public health response to the diseases differs. The rapid spread of the EHF takes place in the hospital setting and among health care providers whilst the spread of HIV is largely within the context of sexual behaviour and practices. Focusing attention on short term preventive measures among health workers is thus a far cry from the long term and sustained effort required for preventive behaviour changes needed for control of the HIV epidemic.

In effect, the distinguishing features of outbreaks and epidemics include the following elements which have significant impact on the health system and public health responses: Outbreaks tend to be localised and of short duration irrespective of their reoccurrence or not. Epidemics tend to be sustained over time and partly as a response, sustained over space. Awareness of outbreaks may be local, but the severity or exotic nature of the disease may result in its sensationalized and global awareness and often response as well. As a result outbreaks can at times attract significant, and to onlookers disproportionate, resources to its control and management. Similarly, the emergence of an epidemic may be incremental and not recognised as such until an elapsed period when the severity, significance and impact of the epidemic is being assessed and debated. This was true of the HIV/AIDS epidemic.

With these distinctions in mind, it is easier to understand why the short term behaviour changes needed for an outbreak can be enforced on the population without the ethical niceties of the informed consent or otherwise of the population. Limitations may be imposed on the movement of people or of agents of transmission of the outbreak which will be impossible in the context of a long term epidemic.

The clarity and logic of the restrictions put in place in an outbreak may be enough justifications for the methods of control. But often the medical and social circumstances fuelling an epidemic may make the imposition of general population control measures difficult to justify. The threat to whole populations in an epidemic is often more selective than the short term threat of an outbreak. In such a situation, the option open to control in an epidemic is to understand the dynamics of the development and progress of the epidemic and design appropriate programmes of behaviour modification and change which contribute to the slowing and elimination of the spread of the epidemic.

From the discussion in this introduction it is apparent that the HIV epidemic requires fundamental changes in basic human beliefs, behaviour and practices in such matters as sexual behaviour, exposure to bodily fluids of infected individuals, as well as the emotional response to those who are infected or affected by the epidemic. Unfortunately, and as will be shown in the next chapter, these sexual and other habits are not easy to change because they are ingrained and have become "habitual".

CHAPTER 2

WHAT ARE HABITS?

INTRODUCTION

Common meaning of habit

The word "habit" is so frequently used that the meaning needs to be clarified in the context of behaviour change. The most helpful definition is that habit is an action or pattern of behaviour that is repeated so often that it becomes typical of somebody, although he or she may not be aware of the action. From childhood one gets used to some adult attempts to correct some of such habits in children: 'Stop picking your nose! 'Do not bite your nails'. The onlooker is aware that it is a habit. The person involved may be unaware that they have the habit until it is pointed out to them.

Habit can also focus on the way something is usually done or routinely done in a particular situation. When the habit is that of a group, it is referred to as custom, that is, something that people in the group always do or always do in a particular way by tradition.

The word "attitude" is often used also to describe habit in terms of somebody's general disposition to things: He or she is too carefree. They are always late to meetings. In effect these attitudes are habitual.

When the habit is in the context of an abuse of substance, then it is termed an "addiction". The habitual use of drugs is one such context. This description of habit is always negative and indicates the helpless submission to an undesirable or damaging habit that the people may or may not be aware of.

In summary, habit is the established pattern of behaviour. It starts off being learnt, then formed into patterns and repeated often enough to become fixed in the mind and in the routine of the individual or group.

Common notion of breaking habits
Given the definitions of habit above and the emerging distinction between habits which may be beneficial or harmful, it is necessary to examine the common notion of how habits can be "broken". The informal phrase "kicking the habit" is used in the context of becoming free of an addiction or stopping something that has been a long standing practice. Another informal phrase which clarifies the process of breaking habits is "turning a new leaf". When people request that some should "reconsider their stand" they are in effect being asked to take into account the information presented to them upon which a wise decision to change their position or habit can be based.

In all of the common notions of breaking habits, there is an implicit assumption that it is the individual or group that has the habit that can change it. This is more than a philosophical idea it is implicit in the legal sense when instructions are given as to which bad habit must go and which must replace it at the risk of a sanction. Wear your seat belt. Do not drink and drive etc., are some of such. But a change of habit can also be imposed through "modifying patterns of behaviour". This is the basis of conditioning in psychology: a method of controlling or influencing the way people or animals behave or think by using a gradual training process. (Microsoft® Encarta® 2009)

WHAT ARE THE ORIGINS OF HABIT?

A number of explanations of the origins of habit have been proposed from various disciplines and insights.

Originates in the learning process

It has been suggested that habit originates in the learning process (Sa Wahid, 2006). According to this approach, the human brain is from birth internally programmed or conditioned through association to recognise pattern of stimulus through the senses of hearing, seeing, touching, tasting and smelling. A pattern is defined as a repeated form of something. When something is repeated frequently enough the brain will recognise it as a pattern. Then the brain will try to associate the pattern with something: either a feeling or a physical/biological response or both. Part of this is what is called the learning process, which also serves partially as safety mechanism for humans as well as other living things when it comes to anticipating danger on the bases of the senses!

Cataloguing of patterns over time

Over time, other patterns are detected and stored to both the conscious and subconscious parts of the mind. In childhood, both the conscious and subconscious minds are flexible and patterns can be changed or modified. But over time the learnt patterns stored in the minds and the responses they elucidate are fixed and the brain becomes inflexible and those things in the mind make up what the individual is.

Fixed habits formed

Once solidified in the mind, the individual will tend to resist vigorously any change which is, in effect, an alteration of learnt patterns. This is how all habits (good or bad) get formed. Once well formed, it becomes next to impossible for most people to change the behaviour and habits.

Language as tool of habit formation

Language plays an important role in the association of patterns. A mention of a fruit [orange, lemon, pawpaw etc] can raise various associations in the mind of the listener in terms of seeing, feeling, smelling and tasting the fruit – all in the mind. Depending on the fruit mentioned, those associations can be pleasant or revolting to the level of prompting an emotional or physical response – salivating, vomiting, hunger etc.
The brain can 'link' events across the senses
Something smelt can be associated with something else we have seen. Something heard can also be linked in the mind with something felt in the past. In effect, all of these cross-referencing are taking place through the medium of the language of the individual even when they are thinking silently (Sa Wahid, 2006).

Habit formed over time

In summary, habits are formed over time and are the result of being repeated enough to become a pattern. They are formed through the use of language, the brain and the senses in the learning process. In other words, habits take time to be fixed and consequently require the right approach and effort to have them changed, if at all possible.

PURPOSE OF HABITS

Once formed habit makes doing things easy

The objective of forming habits is to make doing something easy. The action becomes relatively easy to embark on whereas forcing oneself to perform the action does not last long and is not likely to become habitual. Of course, motivation or willpower which may be defined as a combination of determination and self-discipline enables somebody to do something despite the difficulties involved but it requires constant effort and work to develop the action into a habit. In effect, the goal is to do something long or repeatedly enough until it becomes a habit. Once it becomes a habit, it no longer requires much effort. It becomes automatic.

THREE RELEVANT QUESTIONS

Against the background of the discussion of the formation and purpose of habits so far, there are three questions that arise and need some response. They are:
  Q. 1: Why are habits being classified as being good or bad?
  Q. 2: Why is bad habit retained or so persistent?
  Q. 3: Why adopt a replacing good habit?

Q. 1: Why are habits classified as being good or bad?

A feature of habits is that they become easy to perform irrespective of the moral content and value attached to it. [Any type of habit is relatively easy to develop: the trick is doing it repeatedly enough to become a habit.] The distinction between good and bad habit lies in the moral and value connotations attached to the habit. Bad or undesirable habits [smoking, excessive television viewing, etc.] all have something in common: They all give some type of rewarding feeling to the individual. The rewarding feeling can be relaxation, stress reduction, excitement [adrenalin?] etc. In other words, the reward is independent of the moral value. The anticipation of the reward may become attractive enough to form the basis of addiction. The addiction then is not to the habit but the rewarding feeling. It is this expectation of the "reward" for bad habits that makes individuals continue repeating those habits even after they are aware of the moral content or value attached to the habits. People generally do not do things habitually that makes them feel bad whilst they are engaged in the habit.

Take smoking, the smoker might keep saying they are going to quit after smoking that one cigarette, but during the exercise the mind is focused on the enjoyment and on the state of relaxation. The same goes with the abuse of alcohol. A little feeling of guilt in the back of the mind is subservient to the dominant feeling of enjoyment and hilarity during the process of the drinking.

In contrast to the feeling of reward gained from bad habit, the failure to adopt a "good" habit is because a negative reward is associated with giving up the bad habit or conversely a negative reward is associated with taking up the good habit. Giving up smoking can be associated with the loss of prestige within the smoking fraternity. Giving up unprotected sex can be associated with the loss of "full enjoyment" of the sexual act, etc. To succeed in forming or adopting good habit, a positive reward association must be found for it.

In childhood, finding the good reward for giving up bad habit and presenting it to the child is the parental approach to forming good habits. For example going early to bed may be associated in the mind of the child with loss of privilege, but going to school the next day may be the promised reward for a child who loves going to school. In general it is difficult for children to "wait" for the reward. They find it difficult to focus on the end result in light of the current "enjoyment". Another hour of a favourite television or play time is presenting current reward feeling against which the promise of seeing friend at school the next day pales in significance. They cannot visualize an undesirable outcome of continuing the current line of action.

In contrast to children, responsible adults should be able to form or adopt good habits precisely because they should be able to (a) award the reward soon after taking the good action or have the self discipline to delay reward until later; (b) focus on the end result of taking the good action; and (c) conceptualize the outcome of not taking the good action or performing the good habit.

Q. 2: Why is bad habit retained or so persistent?

At some point, the moral content and value attached to a habit come into focus for the individual or group through exchange of views at different levels. At the level of individuals, the habit elicits reaction on the social, economic, health and other impact. Such impact is either seen as negative, good or indifferent depending on the context in which the habit plays out. Smoking was first stigmatized for its harmful effect on the smoker but as knowledge of the causation of cancer from smoking grew, it became apparent that exposure to the cigarette smoke of others is equally harmful.

The expectation is that when people know the moral content and value attached to the habit that should make it easy or logical for them to make the change in the direction of the good habit. The real problem is that the bad habit is retained on the strength of the "good feeling" of reward associated with it (the issue of addiction may also explain why it is difficult to change behaviour). Conversely, the adoption of the good habit is associated with a loss, a bad feeling, and inferior compensation for the foregoing of the current reward of the bad habit. The current reward of unchanged habit is stronger than an anticipated short and medium term value of the alternate good behaviour. In the throes of a habit, there is either no ability or the ability to think ahead about the values of dropping the habit. Attention needs to be turned to the third question relating to the circumstances for the adoption of a replacing good habit when the bad habit is dropped.

Q. 3: Why adopt a replacing good habit?

If bad habits are retained on the strength of the pleasant feelings or rewards attached to their performance, those bad habits will only be dropped on the strength of the "superior" rewards that can be associated with the adoption of the good habit. The adoption of the good habit is associated with a gain, a good feeling, and superior compensation over and above the current reward of the bad habit. This will happen if there is the ability to "think ahead" in the short and medium term in assessing the positive value of the outcome of changed habit as opposed to the grievous consequences of not changing. It then appears that the change from bad to good habit is substantially cerebral and only partly emotional or spiritual. This has serious implications for behaviour change and its management and orchestration.

Apart from the different perspectives that people bring to their decisions to maintain or change their habits, there are additional complications resulting from the ability of human beings to fake their reactions to behaviour change communications and messages. In addition, people have the capacity to have variations to the extent to which they adopt and apply new habits. A classic example is the selective adoption of safe sex practices such as use of condoms depending on subjective assessment of the risks posed by the sexual partner. Consequently, one of the major challenges of behaviour change communication is to provide sufficient information and guidance upon which people can base more consistent responses.

Pros and cons of bad and good habits

The association of some good feelings to engaging in the good habit is only the beginning. Unlike bad habits, good habits somewhere in the future require focus and work to develop and form. In contrast, the existing bad habits give instant gratification, while developing good habits usually do not. There is usually an opportunity cost of foregoing the reward of the bad habit and the direct cost of adopting the good habit. Consequently, there is often the need for pushing and motivating subject or self to perform the actions to be developed into a habit.

It has to be noted that there are some habits for which the creation of the good feeling is all that is required to make the change. However, for others, it takes effort and some planning before the creation of the pattern of behaviour that becomes the habit can take place

COMMON SENSE APPROACH TO DEVELOPING NEW HABITS

NGO'S 7 STEPS TO DEVELOPING HABITS

Before embarking on an in-depth discussion of the theory and practices of behaviour change, it is worth examining the common sense practical components of changing or modifying behaviour Ngo, (2008) has proposed 7 steps to developing new habits. This framework is one of many but serves the purpose of increasing understanding of the dynamics of habit formation and modification. The seven steps are presented below with some commentary and variations so as to make up for the inherent differences between the society for which the practical processes are proposed and the local circumstances in which behaviour change takes place in Nigeria.

1. [Provide/Have] clear guide on the end result of developing good habits.[including an understanding of the end result of not dropping bad habits]
2. [Provide/Help] Develop strong enough reasons why you want the end result from the good habit.
3. [Provide] Education on what it takes to form [and sustain] the good habit.
4. Prepare [subjects] for attacks on the proposed change to good behaviour.
5. Get reinforcements. [Get ready/Rehearse the counter arguments]
6. Continue on the stairs [Practice] until you reach the escalator [Habit formed].
7. It's all maintenance from here. [Sustain/maintain the new habit]

Although the steps are couched in everyday language, the psychological, intellectual and emotional implications for the subject are profound and need some clarification if the full value of the framework to the modelling of behaviour in traditional and modern populations is to be appreciated. What follows are brief reviews of each of the steps.

Step 1a: Be clear on expected outcome of the good habit including the end result of not changing.

In the context of modern post-industrial societies the responsibility for setting goals may appear to be with the individual. But even in these societies, knowing why one wants to develop the habit in the first place may require the input of policy scientists, researchers and planners. The input is often in terms of prescriptive "do's and don'ts" dictates rather than the result of the personal contemplation of a body of knowledge about the risks and harms attached to a pattern of behaviour or habit.

At the same time as the expected outcome of the new habit is being worked out, the undesirable outcomes of unchanged course of action or habit must also be explained and codified. As with the rationale for the new habit, the source of guidance in an illiterate society is always the elite and the external agents who are not easy to identify with at the community level.

It is worth noting that even health benefits of behaviour change in industrial societies often require the creation of an image in the media for the new objective. Losing weight is as much a health strategy as it is a fashion fad in western countries and through the power of the media, all over the world. The globalization of value is particularly easy and strong among the youth.

But in spite of the normative influence of the media, the consequences of not losing weight still need to be explained to serve as the push factor in the behavioural change process.

Step 1b: End result should be something that excites the individual/group.

Presumably, the creation of excitement is a fixture of modern post-industrial societies. One complication of the HIV/AIDS epidemic is the absence of drama in the causation of the infection. The infective act and knowledge of infection can be separated in time. Consequently, exciting people about improved chances of survival or of escaping a "silent epidemic" is not easy before or after the act.

It is equally difficult to see how a habitual smoker is going to be excited at the chances of longer life at the point of quitting the habit. At the point of death, however, it is likely to be easier to generate regret or remorse of unchanged habit but by then it is too late to alter the course of the outcome of the habit.

Step 2a: Develop strong enough reasons for desiring the 'reward' of good habit

Unfortunately the end results in sexual behaviour change are not contrasted sharply in the mind of people. The alternatives are not dramatic. The sudden post adultery death – *magun* – is an exception in that the link between the adulterous sexual intercourse and the drop dead outcome is direct and dramatic.

Fortunately, there are some graphic materials on the effect of untreated STIs, late stages of AIDS and on the physical and psychological devastation of AIDS on the individual that can form the basis of conversion and commitment to the end result of good habit.

Once the end result is known, identify enough compelling reasons why it is desirable. This is the other side of the coin in developing reasons. The desirability is a factor in the strength of the reasons. The risk of immediate death is a far cry from the risk of eventual death even from the most painful of syndromes including cancers. This is what makes quitting smoking such a burden for some. On the other hand, the money saved from quitting smoking may be attractive enough reason for those with the strength of character to quit for economic reasons.

In the age of graphic illustration of syndromes, the video and images can be powerful tools of explicit illustration of some consequences of habits to convert the audience to alternative habits [e.g. untreated STI and penile decapitation].

Step 2b: Develop Strong Enough Reasons
Most failure to achieve a goal is because the reasons for achieving it were not strong enough to help overcome the setbacks and obstacles. Conversely, the motivation to retain bad habit may be equally or more compelling or the balance of short term pleasure versus long term gain may weaken the resolve to overcome the bad habit. In effect the stronger the reasons for attaining the new habit, the greater the chances of working out any barriers to making the change or in maintaining the new habit.
Some reasons are so compelling that they produce a conversion to the new habit and a strong attachment to the new values and gains associated with it. That process encourages adherence to new habit until it becomes as ingrained as some bad habits are. In the Sexual Reproductive Framework (SRH) the moral beauty of good behaviour is a weaker argument than the raw pleasure of immoral or hazardous sexual habits.

Step 3a: Being educated on preconditions to form and sustain good habit

> *"You've got to know what it really takes. If you go into something blindly, chances are you will be faced with disappointment."*

The challenge of changing behaviour in response to an epidemic is the multiplicity of roles in the process: the infected often do not know they are infected; if they know, they do not know the cause of infection; they may not know the prevention or management of infection.

People who have all the scientific information for prevention and management are often "outsiders to the target population" in terms of socioeconomic status, culture and life style.

To effect the acquisition of knowledge, therefore, a transfer is vital. It is the efficacy of that transfer/communication that is central to "knowing what it takes to form [and sustain] the good habit". The preconditions for practice of good habit until it is ingrained can let converts down in SRH behaviour change.

> *"Let's say your goal is to lose weight. You set a goal to lose 50 pounds in 3 months. Then you work on developing the habit of regular exercise and eating correctly."*

Unlike dietary behaviour the precision of information about sexual behaviour change is not as finely calibrated. Consequently, the burden of educating people for behaviour change in partner reduction, use of condom is lower.

> *"Problem is, you didn't educate yourself enough to know what proper exercising and eating consists of."*

But as with any change of habit educating the target in the ramification of new habit and old habit is the basis on which such other dimensions of change as commitment, perseverance etc. hang.

On the final analysis, the context of new habit including the information, resources and access to them becomes the operational as opposed to intellectual dimension of adopting the new habit and staying with it.

> *"People go to the gym everyday and come home and eat foods they think is healthy. But not knowing what to expect, thinking they had probably lost 15 lbs every month. Two months pass and they've only lost 10 pounds, they always feel tired, and they start to feel discouraged."*

The mechanism of measuring progress indicated for weight loss is relevant to sex behaviour change in as much as there has to be signposts to mark the transition to and formation of new good habit. The target needs competent education/counselling to track the progress they are making and identify the triggers of relapse the better to avoid them.

> *"If educated on proper exercise, dieting, and what to expect, people will feel motivated and energized to keep at it."*

The impression must not be that the sexual behaviour change candidate is passive and needs all stimulus to come from outside. Rather, the counselling process is aimed at getting their first hand knowledge of their strengths and weaknesses to be part of the re-education of the need for change in habit.

Step 4: Reinforcing the new good habits

4a: Prepare for attacks on the proposed change to good

> *"The greatest obstacle you'll face in developing habits will come from your own "gremlins". You know the charming little voice in your head that comes up with about a dozen excuses to not take action. Persuasive little critters they are. Have you ever wanted to develop the habit of waking up at a certain time every morning? You know how it is right? The first few days might be a cinch. But about the end of the first week, you wake up at the right time, but on this day, something wakes up with you and starts a little sales pitch."*

The internal debate is certainly one source of attack on forming new/good habit. But it is not the only one in SRH behaviour change. The internal debate takes place in various moments of choices between two lines of action, each with its own benefits and cost: getting out of bed on a cold morning is often delayed by the inner debate about the costs and benefits of staying in bed. The internal debate takes place on other more serious occasions but has one element in common, that whatever the choice made, there is an accounting of the relative pains and gains of each choice.

Because some of the bad habits were formed in groups at an impressionable period of life, the external sources of attack are particularly important to relapse and lack of commitment. Take allied social bad habits such as smoking, alcohol and drug abuse, multiple sexual partnership; they have some features in common: They are mostly carried out in company and demonstrably to impress and belong in the group. They are no fun unless there is an audience to appreciate the audacity of the habit. There is no such thing as a quiet womanizer. The peers have got to know. At least the confidential womanizer is something of an exception and generally falls outside the teenage and young adult impressionable ages.

4b: Prepare for attacks on the proposed change [Fighting the internal battle]

The greatest threat to sustaining new habits comes from within the individual. It is the product of the continuous internal debate about the gains and losses attached to the new habit. On the one hand, the motivation for making the change is based on an appreciation of the gains from the new habit. However, on the other hand, the memories of the pleasure of the old habit that have had to be given up raise the temptation to relapse. This battle within should be anticipated and prepared for if the gains of new habit are to stay attractive.

The advantage for the subject in fighting the battle is that they know their own weaknesses and their strengths. Carrying out a frequent stock taking of the arguments on either side of the debate will strengthen the resolve to allow the gains to win over the losses attached to lost pleasures of the old habit. Working out how to counter the arguments leading to a relapse can become a useful strategy for overcoming the temptation to go back to the old ways.

4c: Prepare for attacks on the proposed change [Scenario building].

Although the assumption of literacy and associated life style underlies the planning strategy of writing the pro and cons of a line of action down in preparation for tackling attacks on formation of new/good habit. Even illiterates can be mentally equipped through appropriate role play and sharing of experiences during initial training and the follow up sessions which forms an integral part of the new BCC, to prepare their minds for fighting this inner battle. What this training approach does is to prepare the client in anticipatory thinking and mental cataloguing of internal debates won by others and the reasons for failure to overcome what is plainly 'temptation'.

Step 5: Get reinforcements [Get the counter arguments ready].

Box 2.1 shows the prescription of Ngo for this stage of developing new habits. It is presented in full to illustrate the rationality of habit development that is the focus of the Ngo approach. It also illustrates the range of infrastructure available to that rational approach. But the most central issue being raised is the necessity to get ready for the opposition to changing behaviour from others.

Box 2.1

Get Reinforcements

Find ways to remind yourself why you're trying to develop habits. Examples:

Put your goal in writing [and display it] where you can see it every day.

Put a picture of the body you want with your face on it in front of your refrigerator.

Record a message to yourse lf telling yourself why you've got to keep going and listen to it daily.

If you have songs that just pump you up and get you going, listen to them.

Get support from friends and family members to help keep you accountable.

The point of having reinforcements is that it's so easy to get sidetracked from the objective of developing new habits. Having these prompts in front of you every day will remind you of your reasons why you must follow through. It can be conjectured that the longer the period of practice of a new habit the closer it is to making it automatic response. In between the moment of conversion and the forming of the new habit, however, the need for reinforcement comes up periodically and in sympathy with the triggers for going back to the bad habit. If it is alcoholism, every festive occasion raises its challenge. Similarly exposure to friends who are still smoking poses a challenge for someone who has given up smoking. Anticipating the challenges to adhering to new behaviour and planning how to overcome them on basis of past or new experience is the essence of getting reinforced for the event.

If it is promiscuity or having multiple sexual relations that is the changed behaviour, getting psychologically and materially prepared ahead of exposure to risk to relapse makes sense. The psychological preparedness may consist of avoiding the type of friends who encourage promiscuity or obtaining the condom ahead of the potential exposure to unsafe sex which is associated with having multiple sexual partners.

Step 6a: Continue the climb until you reach the plateau

Box 2.2

Get Reinforcements

Find ways to remind yourself why you're trying to develop habits. Examples:

Put your goal in writing [and display it] where you can see it every day.

Put a picture of the body you want with your face on it in front of your refrigerator.

Record a message to yourse If telling yourself why you've got to keep going and listen to it daily.

If you have songs that just pump you up and get you going, listen to them.

Get support from friends and family members to help keep you accountable.

NOT doing it makes you uncomfortable

Prior to the attainment of the habit status, the development stage can be quite demanding. It requires single mindedness to focus on the utility of the new habit without being distracted by the lucre of the old habits. Similarly, the development stage can be quite tedious because it may require new life style to make the performance of the needed task possible and often enough to become the new habit. This aspect of developing a new habit points to the need for an enabling environment which may not be under the control of the subject. This is important in health behaviour change when the adoption of new habit may require that resources, opportunities and facilitating features be in place if the new habit is to be formed and sustained.

Step 6b: Continue the climb until you reach the plateau [Continue on the stairs [Practice] until you reach the escalator [Habit formed]].
Box 2.3

How long does it take to form a habit? Conventional wisdom says 21 − 30 days. It really depends on   the habit from my experience. How long it takes really depends on how fast you can get to the point where it becomes effortless, but for practicality sake, set a goal to do it for at least 30 days, everyday. So your goal is to keep on repeating what you w   ant to develop into a new habit for 30 days so that it becomes a habit.

Regarding the 30 days, know that it's okay to fail. .. *It's not all or nothing* . If 30 days is too long, *break it down* . Do it for 7 days in a row, or 5 days, or 2 days. That's not enough time to form a habit but it will give you confidence that if you can sustain the action for 2 days, you can do it for 5 days and 7 days and so on.

Or you can break it down activity wise . Let's say you want to develop the habit of going to the gym. On da y 4 you stumble. You used everything you could think of but that damn gremlin persuaded you to not go. Instead of beating yourself up, think of a different approach. If going to the gym and working for an hour for 30 days or even 5 days is too much, how ab   out just develop the habit of just going to the gym without actually working out. If that is still too much, how about develop the habit of getting dressed and getting in your car. Now that might sound silly but trust me, it works. Eventually, you'll be si   tting in the car and just think, why don't I just drive to the gym today. Gradually you'll be able to work your way up to actually doing the workout. Keep it simple and take it one step at a time if you have to.

Once you've formed the habit, from this point....

Comments on Stage 6

The key variables at this stage of the Ngo framework are the length of time it takes for a habit to be formed; the possibility of faltering during the habit formation period and starting all over again; and the option of forming the new habit in stages.

On the length of time, it is apparent that some changes to new habits can be on a dramatic basis and that the option of relapse may be closed. Changing from driving on the left side of the road to the right is mandatory. In the early stages of the change over, there might be an occasional memory lapse, but this is quickly corrected on the promptings of other road users or law enforcement officers. The length of time for getting used to a new way of doings things may not be as rigid as road lanes. Consequently, the frequency of performing the new habit will be an influence on the establishment of a pattern of behaviour which may be termed a habit.

But as Ngo points out, there is always the second option of not succeeding at the first try. In such a case, the subject can set intermediate targets for sustaining the new practice and incrementally get to a point of the true formation of the new habit.

The third option which is particularly apt is a systems approach which allows the subject to reach the final objective in stages. An apt example is the quitting of smoking habits. Cutting the number of cigarettes smoked in a day offer such an incremental approach. The assumption is that the staging of the change of habit will reduce the negative impact of quitting "cold turkey" with the attending risk that the reaction of craving for cigarettes may be so overwhelming as to throw the whole project of quitting into danger of collapse.

Step 7: Sustaining/maintaining the new habit
Box 2.4

It's All Maintenance From Here

This is where you want to be at. This is what makes everything easy. ***Once you've developed the habit, it'll no longer be a struggle*** *. You will no longer have to force or motivate yourself to take action. It'll be a part of your life. From here, all you have to do is maintain it. Depending on how strong the habit is,* ***even if you stop say****, going to the gym* ***for a few weeks****, your habit will eventually draw you back*** *into going again. Now and then you might have to* ***get back into a habit of doing something if you've stopped for too long*** *perhaps due to some external circumstances like relocating and not having a gym nearby, but don't worry,* ***the 2nd time around is a lot easier and takes less time.***

Comments on Step 7

Once the habit is formed, it becomes easier to do. Though there might be occasional pauses in performance of the habit, but being a habit it draws the subject back to its performance. But once truly formed, a habit can be resumed even after an elapsed period due to unforeseen circumstances. The resumption is relatively easier than the first attempt at forming the habit because the preparatory steps had already been successfully taken before.

There are of course other practical guides to forming new habits [http://zenhabits.net/7-little-habits-that-can-change-your-life-and-how-to-form-them/], the Ngo framework happens to be the most pertinent of the lot. It is also a useful transitional framework against which to enter the rigorous review of theories of behaviour change in the next chapter. But before then, it is worth mentioning the determinants and co-factors of behaviour change among a traditional society such as the Yoruba. That way, the departures of behaviour formation and change in modern society of the type modelled by Ngo from the traditional counterpart can be fully appreciated.

DETERMINANTS AND CO-FACTORS OF BEHAVIOUR CHANGE AMONG THE YORUBA

Against the background of the pragmatic framework of developing new habits, or by implication changing from a risky behaviour to a health maintaining behaviour, it is worth seeing how these steps fit into the value systems of the Yoruba of Nigeria as well as of other ethnic nations in which behaviour change is a pressing need because of the HIV/AIDS epidemic. Three factors might be cited as having a prominent role in the reception of health risk messages and the adoption of or development of a new pattern of behaviour in such systems. These are the values attached to life or, on the other side of the coin, the fear of death and the fear of shame or loosing face or esteem among peers or in the wider community.

Value of Life
Being alive is one of the greatest resources to the Yoruba. In life is embedded the notion of a better tomorrow. Consequently, holding on to life is considered a priority and threat to life are taken seriously.

Fear of Death
By the fear of death and the desire to propagate and live, the Yoruba's' thoughts were driven to the study in nature of the phenomena that caused death or helped him live and propagate.... "I am wonderstruck that man, governed more or less by his senses and environment should have instinctively built up trains of thought and ways of expressing them that they have led native philosophers to divide their mythology into certain well-defined categories" (Kenneth, 1910 in Agbaje, 2005). Given this fear of death, could this well be an entry point into motivating the Yoruba to good habits with the promise of a longer and healthier life?

Fear of Shame
Among the Yoruba, as in other ethnic groups within and outside Nigeria, it is possible that the fear of shame may on occasions be greater than the fear of death. This social contract is captured in the aphorism "Iku ya ju esin" (better to die than suffer indignity). In effect, the shame of being ridiculed by friends on being informed of sexual behaviour change such as having fewer partners or total abstinence is greater than the future prospect of an uncertain (even if inevitable) death as a result of unchanged habit.

The trouble with psyche at the group or individual level is the subjectivity at the basis of the value position. Some of the subjectivity is to be found in the importance that people attach to hanging on to their dignity even in the face of death. But to be useful, the true cost of death has to be confronted. In the prevailing atmosphere of stigma attached to HIV infection at the start of the epidemic, the fact that such infection is survivable alters the basis of fear of death and shame of being known to have died from HIV infection. In other words, there are occasions when death itself is the greater shame.

The way to tipping the balance between shame of ridicule and unnecessary death that brings posthumous ridicule is to place both shame and death in reasoned rather than normative response to behaviour change. The solution is to be found in another Yoruba philosophical position when the need to turn to a new behaviour is so universal as to negate any sense of shame at being ridiculed or any loss of dignity. This is the situation that prompts the saying among the Yourba – "orun nya bo ki se oro eni kan", literally translated as "that the heavens are falling down is not an individual disaster." In effect the common destiny makes an eventuality, however unpleasant, that much more acceptable and can help overpower any lingering sense of individual shame.

Soon after the "disaster" a sense emerges that any change which it entails becomes the new norm, that is, if the society or community is to survive the disaster. When the change becomes normative through its common community level adoption then it is easier to change without a sense of shame. Prior to the normative state of the new reality, it is the secrecy attached to individual choices that obscures the rapid emergence of normative behaviour. Finding a way of breaking the taboo or code of secrecy may be a precondition to recognition of the normative value of an emerging new pattern of behaviour.

Box 2.5

The natural urge and aspiration for freedom took over the psyche of Nigerians between 1993 and 1998 leading to the most consistent and persistent struggle against oppression in general and against military dictatorship in particular. It yielded an outcome in 1999 with the return to civil administration. Yet it soon turned out again that the captivity wasn't over; that those engaged in the struggle against the military got involved for different purposes and different agenda. For the few that have always had their gaze set on exploiting the system, it was an agenda of impoverishing the people and rendering them subservient, that is, captive. The people are still at the mercy of a few. The story has not changed. This is where we are now.

It is not an unusual story. It is the human story. Indeed we only kid ourselves when we nostalgically refer to the pre-colonial story of our forebears as flawless. They had their encounters with the dark side of humanity. But they were not docile accomplices to the crime of greed and avarice. Each protected his space and family to the best of his ability. That was what chivalry was about. Iku ya j'esin: better to die than suffer indignity. That spirit moderated the aggression of others.

The nation's story of the captivity of the many by the few and the frustration of dreams which it entails is a betrayal of trust. It will not change until the captives took a firm decision followed with a deliberate action to take back their life and their freedom.

[http://thenationonlineng.net/web3/columnist/friday/segun-gbadegesin/12762.html]

COST OF CHANGE: SOCIAL, PSYCHOLOGICAL AND ECONOMIC

As in other societies and populations, the Yoruba also have an accounting of the cost of change which needs to be factored into designing a behavioural change model which will feed into such accounting system. At the social and psychological levels, habits play a vital role in self esteem and in the valuation of what others are supposed to think of one – the peer at any time of life are made up of those whose opinions/views one values. Being an accepted member of the peer group attracts some tangible and intangible privileges. Changing behaviour may risk the loss of those privileges in the social group to which one belongs. Such a loss is very difficult for the Yoruba to handle given the importance attached to social group membership in life and to the favours which such membership can attract even after death.

Apart from the social and psychological benefits of conformity, the economic or opportunity costs of changing behaviour can also be very high. One of the outcomes of group membership to which we alluded is that such groups become a "cooperative" in dealing with individuals' economic, social and spiritual problems. The redistribution of resources is an essential part of that cooperative. In addition, actual monetary contributions may be made by group members in anticipation of providing a pool for times of need by members. Consequently, there is a direct economic cost of loosing acceptance in groups and being excluded from some of these economic benefits.

The group members can also serve as a clientele base from which individuals can draw patronage for their economic activities. Members can also provide a network of patronage with other groups to which they belong. That expansion of network can only subsist when the individual still enjoys the acceptance of the group.

Quite apart from the social, psychological aspects and impact of loosing group membership is the moral and spiritual value that individuals attach to a given pattern of behaviour and to the implications of changing to a new pattern. But the moral valuation can be distorted by the preference of the group. If being a promiscuous person is the norm in a social group, then the idea of partner reduction by a member is considered disloyal to the group value. Consequently, the valuation of a previous and a new behaviour may tilt the balance against making the behaviour change irrespective of the health and other benefits of the change.

The benefits of not changing

As in other populations too, habits are formed by the Yoruba in the first instance to satisfy a "felt need" – sex, acceptance, esteem, or plain hedonism! To make a change is to have a new need established which meets the test of the social, psychological and economic costs. Because of the nature of habits though, the duration of the existing habit can act as a drag on making the change. An inverse relation develops between length of habit time and probability of making a switch. And a converse inverse relationship can be postulated between time and effort: the longer the habit has been in place, the greater the effort needed to 'break' it. These relationships exist because habit is normative and making a decision to change becomes stressful.   In effect, change is the outcome of sequence of events which has to be structured if the goal of change is to be achieved. That structure benefits from an appreciation of the innate characteristics of the people but gains legitimacy from an appreciation of the theory of behaviour change as postulated elsewhere and only subject to limited application in local populations, that is, beyond the frequent but limited "proof of concept" which most health education experimental interventions amount to. Consequently, attention is turned to a review of existing theories and models of behaviour change in the next chapter.

CHAPTER 3
REVIEW OF EXISTING THEORIES
AND MODELS OF BEHAVIOUR CHANGE

CONCEPTUAL PRECONDITIONS OF BEHAVIOUR CHANGE

There are four possible stages from the awareness of a health risk to the changing of behaviour and practices needed to eliminate or modify the risk. Understanding the stages is a function of the level of sophistication, exposure to information and the ability to process the information. Making the needed changes is a function of the awareness of one's vulnerability and the access to the resources and personal authority/power to take the necessary decisions and put them into action in changing behaviour from the risky one to a non- or less risky form.

In the course of the past century and especially after the Second World War, organisation dynamics and public health practitioners have attempted to find the theories and practices of behaviour change that best explain conditions in their populations and societies of study. Populations and societies however vary as to sophistication, media penetration and other pre-conditions of behaviour change.

Objectives of the chapter
In this chapter we will present a brief review of existing theories that have been largely developed for modern societies and find out how they are relevant to the situations in pre-modern or so called traditional societies. It is in the context of this review that we will shape a 4-stage framework that best fits the Nigerian (Yoruba) sociological context and upon which the intuitive HIV prevention activities on APIN/ARFH project have been based in the past decade (2000 to 2009.

As will be shown, the socioeconomic status of people, their world view, the cultural values they hold and their ability to process modern scientific information speedily and act on such information sets post industrial society apart from traditional societies in developing countries. These differences need to be the basis of the adoption or adaptation of received theories to the local situation in the process of behaviour change communication and engineering.

In that review attention will focus on the role of effective risk or vulnerability assessment carried out on one's own or with assistance from competent facilitators and upon which the individual's engagement with the process of behaviour change is based.

REVIEW OF EXISTING THEORIES

There are five theories and modelling of behaviour change which have been included in this chapter as being the most relevant to the issues of cultural context and sophistication of a society if effective behaviour change communication is to take place. They are Change Process developed by Kurt Lewin (1936, 1947, 1953); Theory of Reasoned Action based on the work of Martin Fishbein and Icek Ajzen (1975, 1980); Health Belief Model (HBM) developed by Ross and Mico (1980) and expanded by Graeff, Elder and Booth (1993), the Social Learning/Cognitive Theory developed by Albert Bandura largely in response to the HIV/AIDS epidemic (1982, 1988), and the Stages of Change developed by Prochaska, DiClemente, and Norcross, (1992).

Whilst the theories emerged from different situations they share their American/European Western background and their adaptation to modern societies in common. Most of the theorists point out this culture specificity in their work (Essien et al., 2005). But the emphasis in the review process is to identify those elements that are most pertinent to the construction of the indigenized 4-Stage process of change within Yoruba society in which it has so far been tested and proven and with possible application to similar pre-modern societies in Nigeria and elsewhere.

[1]   CHANGE PROCESS [Lewin, 1953]

In both chronological and intellectual terms the Change Process developed by Lewin (1936, 1947 & 1953) forms the point of departure to the application of systems thinking and modelling to health behaviour collectively described as Health Belief Models (HBM). An early model of change developed by Lewin described change as a three-stage process.

The first stage he called "unfreezing". It involved overcoming inertia and dismantling the existing "mind set". For this to be achieved, the defence mechanisms that have been in place to prevent change have to be bypassed. In the second stage the change occurs. This stage is typically a period of confusion and transition. The individual is aware that the old ways are being challenged but does not have a clear picture as to what it will be replacing those old ways yet. The third and final stage he called "freezing". In this period, the new mindset is crystallizing and the subject's comfort level is returning to previous levels experienced with the old habits. This is often misquoted as "refreezing" (see Lewin (1947, Frontiers in Group Dynamics)). It should be borne in mind that the ideals of Lewin addressed organisations and group dynamics as well as individual behaviour change.

Lewin's Equation

The famous Lewin's equation $B=f(P,E)$, is a psychological equation of behaviour which states that behaviour (B) is a function of the person (P)and their environment (E)

(Lewin, 1936 in Sansone, Morf & Panter, 2003). This equation is the psychologist's most well known formula in social psychology, of which Lewin was a modern pioneer. It explains the manner in which the personality, attitudes, motivation and behaviour of the individual influence, and are influenced by, social groups. This also includes the attribution of social status based on perceptual cues, the influence of social factors (such as peers) on a person's attitudes and beliefs, the functioning of small groups and large organisations, and the dynamics of face to face interactions The innovation was that Lewin's theory gave importance to a person's momentary [short term] situation in understanding their behaviour, rather than relying entirely on the past as other theories tended to do (Balkenius, 1995).

Figure 3.1: Lewin's 3 Stage Model

Phase	Action
① Unfreeze	Create initial motivation to change by convincing people that current state is undesirable.
② Change	Identify new behaviours and norms. Communicate. Adopt new attitudes and culture.
③ Refreeze	Reinforce new behaviour through reward systems, communications, structures etc.

Source: K. Lewin, Field Theory in Social Science, Harper and Row, 1951. This diagram has been recreated by LMC. [www.lmcuk.com/management-tool/lewins-3-stage-model - Cached]

Implications of Lewin's Change Process

The first obvious implication is that the change process to a new behaviour involves a series of steps which has been further elaborated as [Unfreeze $\rightarrow$ Evaluate $\rightarrow$ Goal Setting $\rightarrow$ Trial/action $\rightarrow$ Refreeze]. By the same token, knowing the forces in favour or against moving from step to step forms the basis of helping people change behaviour. In effect, there is the need to study the societal, organisational or contextual setting prior to engineering change.

Another implication is that Lewin's un-Freeze & re-Freeze model with which habitual behaviour is given up and new/alternative ones are adopted often require new skills, knowledge and social support to help make the change and sustain it over time. In effect, Lewin has set the stage for the review of other theories and point to the need to continually fit theories to the reality of behaviour change situations rather than push reality to fit theories that are often developed in different social, cultural and economic settings. [This is of tremendous help to developing country scientists who often find that the context in which they operate contains situations that distort the theoretical framework or make a wholesale application of the theory impracticable.

[2]   THEORY OF REASONED ACTION [Martin Fishbein and Icek Ajzen, 1975, 1980]

This theory is also known as Theory of Planned Behaviour and has 3 components:
The first is the attitude toward the behaviour. This is based on the view or perception that performing the behaviour will lead to certain outcomes and the evaluation of these outcomes are considered as favourable or otherwise.

The second are the subjective norms which take into account the influence of relevant others in one's social environment or network on the behavioural intentions. The greater the respect attached to those others' opinion, the greater their influence on the subjective norms.

The third component is the intentions to perform the behaviour on the premise that the intentions can be predicted from the combined effect of attitude and subjective norms regarding the action.

Remarks on TRA/TPA

On the basis of these components some comments can be made as to the fit of the TRA/TPA to conditions prevailing in pre-industrial society such as found in Nigeria. As most western scholars will agree, the behaviour change theories (BCT) were developed in industrial societies in which the organisation, environment and individual circumstances relevant to health related behaviour change are radically different to those obtaining in pre-industrial societies such as found in Nigeria. Consequently, there are compatibility problems in the wholesale adaptation of those theories when they are being tested or adapted for interventions elsewhere. In each of the three elements of the TRA/TPA therefore, there are some elements of such imperfect fits.

Imperfections in TRA/TPA fit: Attitude toward the behaviour

The ability to form views on outcomes, and evaluate such outcomes as positive or negative is a function of the sophistication of the message, the sender and the receiver [$Fv=f(Sm, s, r)$. For example, if a correct message comes from a wrong messenger this can lead to the message being tainted in the eye of the receiver and generate an unfavourable reception. Similarly, the knowledge base of the receiver upon which the message and its evaluation are being grafted can influence the evaluation of outcomes. If there is the body of knowledge within which the message can be comprehended, then the chances of the outcomes being correctly evaluated are higher than if otherwise. Revisiting the knowledge base and updating it may be the only reiteration that can lead to competent evaluation of outcomes. In illiterate populations the communication and evaluation of outcomes of scientific and medical events requires that attention be paid to this imperfection in the knowledge base of the target population if the fit of theory to practice is to be improved. The most pertinent of those imperfections such as the comprehension of concepts of viruses, microbes etc., affects both the illiterate and even the educated. The difference is that those who are educated can derive parallel concepts from other domains to help clarify the message.

Imperfections in TRA/TPA fit: Subjective perception of norms

Although people all over the world are sensitive to other's opinion of them, the objective or subjective basis of such opinions depends on a range of communication issues which firmly set the sophisticated societies apart from the traditional. The objectivity of such opinions are influenced by such personal characteristics as education level, exposure to the range of information and the skills needed to make an informed and objective opinion. In contrast, the social and cultural values people hold and the prejudices they have about phenomena influence the way people interpret the information they have. Consequently subjective opinions can in fact be based on factual information. Worse still, when prejudices are combined with inadequate information, then the chances of opinions held being fallacious increases. In the realm of health related behaviour, if the peoples' opinions are based on wrong notions of the causation of health and associated behavioural issues, then the intention to perform a given behaviour on the basis of such notions is flawed.

It is only when there has been a saturation of appropriate information and the homogenisation of understanding of issues in the target population that the reliability of the opinions they hold of a particular behaviour can truly form the valid basis of presuming the intention to perform a given behaviour.

To illustrate, if HIV infection is conceived by relevant others as caused by evil spirit, then changing sexual behaviour in response to the epidemic will not make sense to those others and the change might be conceived as grounded in other interpersonal issues. It is this misfit between the new paradigm upon which the subject based behaviour change and the old paradigm held by relevant others that has to be taken into greater consideration in traditional societies in the process of behaviour change.

Imperfections in TRA/TPA fit: Intentions to perform the behaviour

The predictive value of attitude and subjective norms on intentions to make changes in behaviour is not in doubt once the basis of the perjured assessment of changed behaviour by relevant others have been taken into account. Otherwise, the predictive power of the two elements will be compromised to the extent to which the attitudes were imperfect and the norms based on different world view and understanding of biomedical events.

Finally, the TRA/TPA stops short of tackling the power relations and dynamics between actors in behaviour change which are fundamental to the eventual translation of intention into practice. For example, sexuality is often dyadic behaviour. Consequently, the reactions of others such as sexual partners, society, marital status and the power relations and hierarchy in social, economic and cultural settings will affect the implementation of intentions. The field of family planning is populated by unattained intentions to act on various aspects of family formation and population control. This power dynamics is well illustrated in HIV prevention by condom use which has to be placed in a negotiating context if it is to happen. This omission is taken care of in Health Belief Model.

Two options are open to developing country scientists in their attempt to address the impact fit of theory in real life situations. First, they can, at the risk or not being published "panel-beat" the theory to fit their own setting and hope that methodological rigour will save the situation. Secondly, they can, as often is the case "tailor" the conditions of the intervention to the limitations imposed by the theory. When this alternative is adopted it can constrain the richness of options within the intervention and reduce the practical contributions to such a level that such interventions are essentially proof of concepts rather than a full application and concomitant testing of theory.

For example, prior to the current HIV/AIDS epidemic in Nigeria, health education interventions focused on short term health behaviour change so as to be able to demonstrate the responsiveness of the target populations to the messages or concepts to which they have been exposed in the course of a project (Oladipo, 2002; Nwadigwe 2012). But often the changes registered in the very short term do not stand the test of time and reveal the imperfections in the materials and methods of such interventions largely based on Western models.

[3] HEALTH BELIEF MODEL [Ross and Mico, 1980; Graeff, Elder, Booth, 1993]

According to HBM, health related behaviour is determined by whether individuals:
a. Believe that they are susceptible to a particular health problem;
b. Regard the problem as serious;
c. Convinced that treatment or preventive action are effective/And at the same time inexpensive;
d. Receive a prompt to take health action.

(a) Recognition of health problems and susceptibility

Needless to say, the true recognition of a health problem [as opposed to the mythical recognition] is precondition for appreciation of susceptibility. In knowledge of hindsight, the appearance of the syndrome that became HIV/AIDS among homosexuals led to the assumption that those who are heterosexual are safe from the epidemic! Without belabouring the modern/traditional society dichotomy, the ability of modern societies to recognise health problems is not infinite and some health hazards are unknown to science much earlier before they begin to wreak havoc on the population. The HIV and AIDS pandemic also is a case in point. The advent and management of transient global epidemics demonstrate that the pathway to health behaviour change is not as sequential and coherent as theory would like to make it.

In less developed countries, therefore, both the recognition of health problems and the determination of susceptibility become the primary responsibility of public health practitioners and only then are these conveyed in health interventions to the target population in a form, sequence and circumstances that make the other conditions of behaviour change discussed so far tenable.

(b) Determination of seriousness of health issue

In as much as the identification, much less, seriousness of [some public] health issue is beyond most people in traditional and non-literate society and even in parts of the population of modern societies, the determination of the seriousness becomes a state function handled often by highly trained scientists. Bird flu, mouth and foot disease, HIV and other recent epidemics are primarily identified and assessed as serious by these experts. They too determine other elements such as effectiveness and cost before it becomes the public health tool for the control of the epidemics. The communication of that health issue and its seriousness to the larger population is the starting event in the chain reaction otherwise known as behaviour change.

It is worth noting that in response to the circumstances of the HIV/AIDS epidemic efforts have been made in addressing some of the limitations of the HBM (Rosenstock I., Strecher, V., and Becker, M., 1994). In Figure 3.2 the factors of behaviour change are regrouped into three, namely, the background factors or the determinant of change. These are largely demographic and socio-economic variables which can condition the positions one takes about phenomena. This is followed by perception variables which are either expectations based on benefits, obstacles to action and the capacity one has to take the action. The final set are the action variables which include the cue to action and the actual behaviour aimed at risk reduction or modification if the expectations and threats are to be addressed by the individual.

Figure 3.2: Framework for Behaviour Change – Health Belief Mode

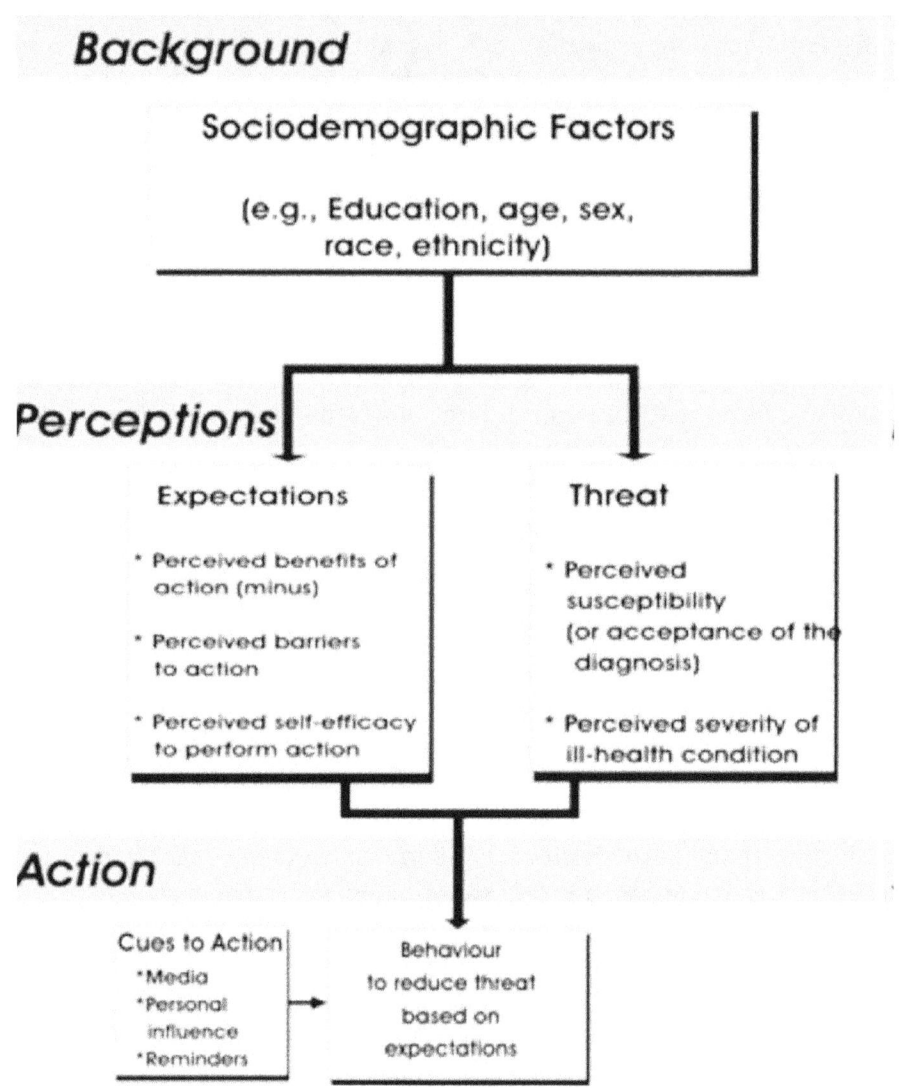

(c)   Effectiveness and cost of treatment/action

When attention turns to the effectiveness and cost of action in pre-modern societies, the conflict between the two can be a conscious barrier to inaction. In the first instance, the determination of the effectiveness and cost of treatment is nearly always located in industrial world where the health problem may not be an issue but where the profit motive is often the driving motive for innovation in health research.   On the other hand, effective treatment may be costly on account of the scale of demand and the high cost of research and development of such treatment.

Even in low technology solutions, the effectiveness of treatment may carry an indirect cost that the subject is unwilling to assume. For example, boiling water to prevent water borne diseases which occur cyclically in poor population is a classic demonstration that the decision to not take action can be plainly logical in light of the prohibitive cost of fuel in any form, including firewood, in developing societies. Often though, the costing of treatment or health solution is short term and may be unaware of the medium to long term cost effectiveness of the solution. However, innovative approaches to the communication of the short, medium and long time costs of inaction can make preventive action or treatment attractive even in a poor population.

By the same token, the subsidy of treatment for HIV-related conditions reduces the burden of behaviour change to demonstrating the effectiveness of treatment to the population in a form, usually through role modelling or interpersonal communication that is easily comprehended even in a non-literate population. In this context, the scaling up of HIV treatment is both a function of price reduction and of the increasing demonstration to the public that with treatment, HIV infection is manageable and survivable. Often the treatment access comes before the demonstration effect.

(d)   Receive prompt/cue to take health action

In health seeking behaviour for example, the cues to action include events, bodily experience (symptoms) of a health condition or environmental circumstances (media publicity) that motivate/push people to take action in a desired direction. It has been pointed out that this aspect of the HBM has not been systematically studied. There is an obvious problem with this element of the HBM. The cue(s) to action might well be the first element of a chain of events, that is, the identification of the health problem and not the last element when all the seriousness, vulnerability and efficacy of treatment issues have been taken into account.

The medial publicity surrounding the advent of a new disease and description of symptoms to watch out for can be ignored if the personal vulnerability has not been determined by the individual. It is only after that determination that the issue of effective and inexpensive treatment or cost of action can become issues. These issues of sequence of event in the process of change and the cause and effect relationships that need to be established is clarified in the next set of theories to be reviewed.

[4]   SOCIAL LEARNING/COGNITIVE THEORY [Bandura, 1982, 1988]

Basic concepts
There are six basic concepts underpinning SL/CT that need to be endowed with meaning the better to understand the operation of the process of social learning:
   a.   Reciprocal Determinism = dynamic interactions of the person, behaviour and environment
   b.   Environment = factors physically external to the person and the opportunities

for social support
c. Observational learning is from actions and outcomes of others' behaviour within the environment
d. Self efficacy = person's confidence in performing a particular behaviour
e. Expectations = anticipated outcomes of behaviour, and
f. Expectancies = the values a person attaches to a given outcome

A rider is that Self-Efficacy increases through information, modelling and practice so that the equilibrium of the decision process can be maintained in the mind of the subject.

Comments on basic concepts

Against the background of the specification of the other theories, Bandura (1982, 1988) within the context of the HIV/AIDS epidemic puts some order into the formulation by providing the explicit concepts and their meanings. In the same way as Lewin, interaction with others and the environment is given important consideration in the modelling. The role of others in the formation of ideas and acquisition of skills is added to the mix. Consequently, the assessment of outcomes is now related to the value systems to which the individual ascribes. Armed with these concepts it is easy to establish cause and effects in a much more detailed way than in the other theories. A number of such schematic presentations of the model are presented below based on Ajzen's Theory of Reasoned Action.

Schematic presentation of proximate determinants of new behaviour

Figure 3.3 shows that in the proximate determinants framework, the new behaviour is the expected outcome. The three variables serve as the proximate determinants of that new behaviour: without them there will be no new behaviour or outcome. But these determinants are themselves outcomes of other variables which are in effect background variables to the proximate ones.

Figure 3.3: Schema Presenting the Proximate Determinants of New Behaviour

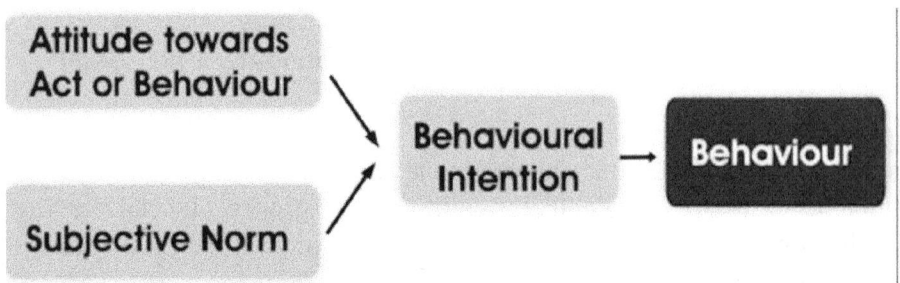

Schematic presentation of the background variables

In Figure 3.4 a pair of background variables determines each of two proximate variables. For Attitude they are beliefs about the behaviour and evaluation of the behaviour as positive or negative. For subjective norm they are opinion of referent others and the motivation to comply.

Fig. 3.4 Schematic presentation of the background variables (Theory of Reasoned Action)

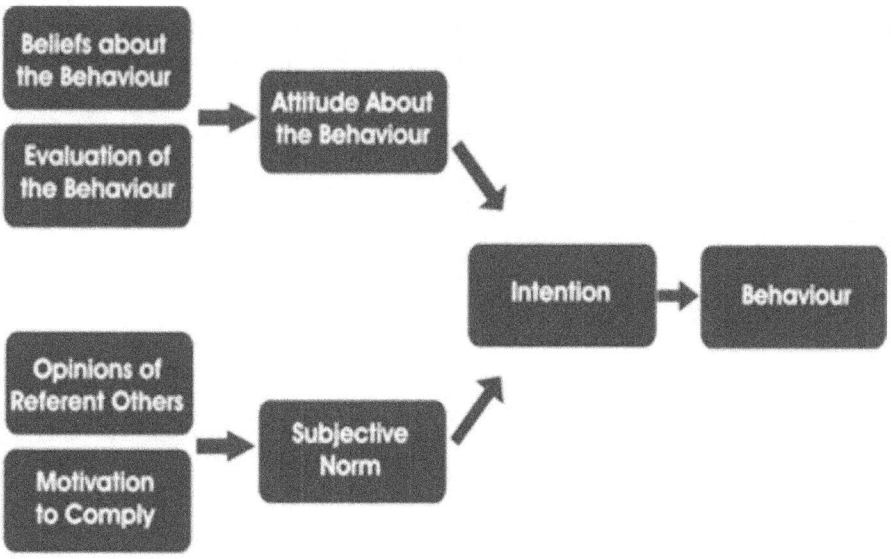

Fishbein-Ajzen Theory of Reasoned Action

Further clarification of the background variable (Strobe, 2000)

As pointed out in the review of the TRA/TPA, belief about the outcome is either based on the ability to make informed assessment of the evidence presented or it can be based on faith or trust of the judgment of others. The evaluation of the outcome as desirable is a function of the level of making comparative analysis of statuses. This can also be taken on trust.

The role of normative beliefs is particularly strong in traditional, communal groups. But reliance on "experts" is also a safety valve with which they cope with their limited capacity to evaluate scientific evidence. Since the modern explanation of disease outbreaks employs some concepts that are foreign to the native population, a leap of faith is often required in the population if they are to accept those explanations. That leap is required because some of the causes and effects proposed by the experts cannot always be demonstrated in the physical realm or in operational terms that makes sense to the general population.

Take the case of water purification as a way of reducing outbreaks of cholera for example: not only is the physical appearance of water not enough basis for assuring its purity, the practical experiences of the local population may involve their use of unclean water without any demonstrable negative impact on their lives, at least in the short run. In such circumstances unquestioning acceptance of modern scientific explanation may be required as an input into effecting behaviour change.

Water from the local stream may be clearer than the water from the public water system. But, without a test for purity of the local stream, there is no telling what diseases may be caused by drinking from the local stream, without boiling first. Such string of argument raises both practical and logistics problems. The immediacy of need for water may make the logic of boiling to attain purity unacceptable. And the cost of purification may also make adherence to the scientific guideline untenable.

Figure 3.5: Further clarifications about background variables by Strobe (2000)

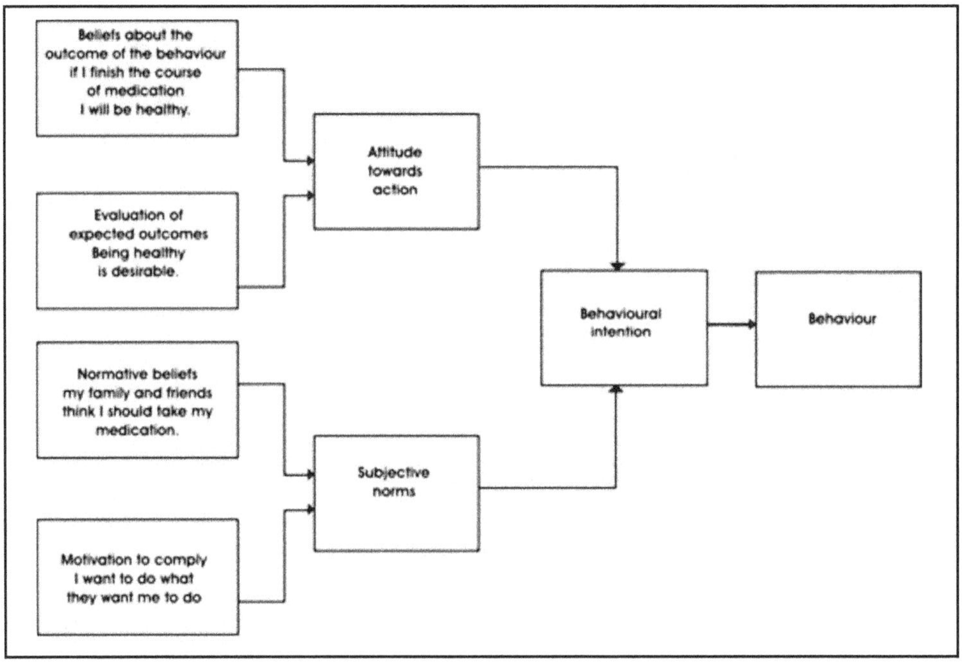

Adapted from Strobe, 2000

[5] STAGES OF CHANGE

In addressing the changing of addictive behaviour Prochaska et al. (1992) applied the stages of change which in effect reflect the sequence of events surrounding the formation of ideas about health problems in terms of recognition, assessing vulnerability and reviewing the efficacy, cost and chances of taking control of the situation. These stages are shown schematically in Table 3.6 below.

Figure 3.6: Stages are shown schematically

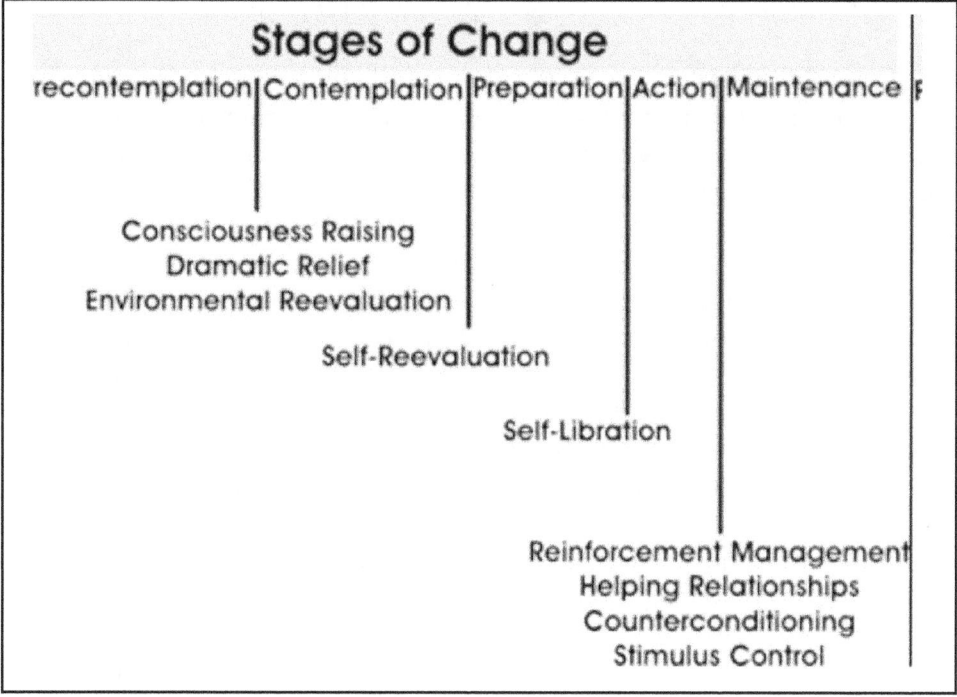

Source: Prochaska, DiClemente and Norcross, 1992.

Comments on stages of change

In the context of the HIV/AIDS epidemic, and in pre-literate societies, the significance of each of the stages and their relevance to BCC are critical to the adaptation of the theoretical and modelling formulations to local conditions in Africa and Nigeria. First, the pre-contemplation stage appears logical starting point or aspect of health related behaviour. However, there is an assumption of a period of total ignorance of a health situation prior to the consciousness raising event that forms the basis of contemplation rather than pre-contemplation. This is true of the Los Angeles gay community prior to the alarm about cases of Kaposi's sarcoma and the eventual recognition of the new syndrome. It is also still true of most of the Nigerian population who have "heard of AIDS" without any appreciation of the true import of the HIV infection and the role it plays in the epidemic.

Against the limitations of access and comprehension of health information made available through any communication medium, the minimum conditions for "encountering" or entering the stages of consciousness raising and contemplation of the epidemic are as follows: either exposure to comprehensive and well packaged mass media communication or participation in a group health talk by a well trained and competent outreach agent or involvement in an equally competent one-on-one counselling within the VCT clinic. A well planned programme of multimedia communication to peer educators in the training setting is aimed at equipping them and empowering them to provide the communication package upon which their contacts can base the process of change or the stages of change.

In effect, the ability to access and comprehend the information is enhanced if BCC implementers bring together a range of information upon which the act of recognition of the health hazard as well as a preliminary assessment of personal or group vulnerability can be based. It is clear from the Change Process that the societal, organisational and contextual setting is always in a flux and that these settings are not the same from one society to another and that there could be variations within a nation. In traditional society, the variety of ethnic nations also implies a variety of settings that must be taken into consideration in understanding or engineering change. What TRA/TPB does is to draw attention to the cause and effect analysis that goes into each change. It takes the competing interests of the subject into account in the process of decision making as to which line of action to take. The TRA/TPB takes the predictive element of change into perspective by linking attitude and subjective norms to the intentions to perform the behaviour. Whilst this predictive value can be articulated with some precision in modern societies, the imperfections of the traditional/pre-modern society can distort that precision.

In the case of HBM, the mechanism of change process is more clearly articulated so that each next step is conditional upon the analysis of the previous stage. But as has been pointed out above, HBM specifications pose a great challenge to interventions in pre-modern populations. The imperfections in the understanding of scientific phenomena, the existence of alternative belief systems and the inadequacies of local languages to cope with health related explanations all combine to make some modification to the specifications and the operational details of health interventions in such populations. It should be emphasized that these limitations of the pre-modern populations are not evidence of intellectual inferiority but setbacks which can be overcome when the limitations have been recognized for what they are.

Under these circumstances, therefore, the researcher carries substantial responsibility for the tailoring of the change to the circumstances and limitation of the population in such a way as to increase the probability of appropriate change taking place. Nonetheless, such tailoring must be within the confines of ethical considerations and acceptable academic and intellectual standards. An example of such ethical issue is to translate scientific phenomenon in such a way as to frighten rather than inform the audience of the actual probabilities they face in any given situation. When such scare tactics are based on the imperfect understanding of the phenomenon as it unfolds, there is not ethical breach. This was the case with the initial stage of HIV prevention tactics in the 1980s and 90s when the "killer disease" image of the HIV/AIDS epidemic was forged. The unfortunate outcomes which were later to complicate HIV prevention and management strategies include the stigmatization of persons living with HIV/AIDS and the fear of taking an HIV test which was seen as receiving a death sentence if one tested positive. It explains why the progress in ART programmes can be linked with the demonstrable effectiveness of such therapies and the realization that early detection is a vital part of that survival strategy.

In the case of Bandura's Social Learning/Cognitive Theory the process of change is more roundly placed in the interaction of the person, their environment, and their self efficacy which in turn interacts with the information for change, the modeling of new behaviour and practice of same until the subject is comfortable with making and sustaining the change. Modifications of the SL/CT by others emphasize the channels of determination of behaviour and clarify the preconditions for every element of change.

QUESTIONS ARISING FROM THE REVIEW

There are four operational questions that can be raised on the basis of the preceding reviews. Why change behaviour? When is behaviour changed? And how is behaviour changed? How can change in behaviour be sustained?

Q. 1 Why change behaviour?

The three major reasons for changing behaviour include the recognition of a desired outcome or fear of an undesirable outcome if behaviour is not changed; the recognition or acceptance that the benefits outweigh the costs of changing behaviour; and an assessment of how relevant others feel about one changing or not changing behaviour.

Q. 2: When is behaviour changed?

Behaviour is changed when the knowledge base upon which the change process will be based has been accumulated. The skill for new behaviour also has to be acquired before the change can take place. In addition the resources for adopting new behaviour will need to be available to make change possible. Furthermore, the individual must be convinced that change is will be of personal benefit. And finally, the physical or social support environment for the new behaviour has to be created before change can happen.

Q. 3: How is behaviour changed?

Anyone who has stopped a long standing habit such as smoking will be aware that there are different methods adopted in the process of changing behaviour. Some have the ability to go through a dramatic change in which there is a sudden termination of old behaviour and the immediate commencement of new behaviour. This may be described as a process of conversion.

For others, the dramatic is inconceivable and change has to be in transitions. This transitional approach involves the modification of behaviour from more hazardous to less hazardous over time. For example, the reduction of number of sticks of cigarette consumed per day over time as a way to terminating smoking is a familiar transitional example of behaviour change (use of modification of behaviour in HIV will also be useful; e.g. use of condom instead of abstinence.

Q 4. How can change in behaviour be sustained?

Sustaining new behaviour as pointed out earlier depends on a number of factors. Is the new behaviour grounded enough to have become a habit? Are there occasions when circumstances in one's environment draw attention and interest in old habits? In other words, is the social environment supportive enough of the new pattern of behaviour? The answer to these questions of sustainable behaviour lies in the strength of character that the individual brings to the new behaviour.

Making the initial change is indicative of some character, but unanticipated consequences of changing behaviour may raise doubts and shake one's confidence. The ability to sustain the new habit inevitably has a spiritual element. If the individual is not fully convinced about the seriousness of consequences of action or inaction then backsliding into old habits can be tempting.

INTUITIVE STAGED BEHAVIOUR CHANGE

Planned change, whether theory based or intuitive, provides a comprehensive manipulation of behaviour by addressing the Why, When, and How? The manipulation can take all three questions together or in some sequence depending on the target, the behaviour and the prevailing learning circumstances. The ultimate purpose is to make sure that the new behaviour is maintained over time so as to attain the goal of the behaviour change communication such as HIV prevention and control. This was the experience on the ARFH/APIN HIV Prevention Initiative in Oyo State that spanned a period of more than 10 years starting from 2001. The contributions of projects executed under the initiative to the emergence of the intuitive staged behaviour change are substantial. They also form the illustrative material presented in Part 2 of this book as to how the validity and robustness of the staged behaviour change developed from sub-project to sub-project.

One feature of the theories and models reviewed is that the locus of control of all phases is largely with the individual. This is possible because of the knowledge base and personal characteristics that the individual starts with in the process of health behaviour change. It is possible to pre-contemplate as Prochaska et. al., (1992) suggest, if one is literate, has an ongoing contact with various media and has a modern biological framework for disease causation and management.

Similarly, the control of the subjective norm on individual behaviour in a community is likely to be in inverse relationship with the strength of those norms. When norms are strong and individuals are weak or lack knowledge base on which to make independent decisions, then the norms prevail. And vice-versa when norms are weak and individuals are empowered by social and economic status they are able to ignore the norms and innovate.

In the next chapter, a 4-Stage Intuitive Model of Behaviour Change derived from 10 years of HIV prevention activities on an ARFH/APIN project illustrates how the received theories and models have been significantly modified and adapted to the circumstances in southwest Nigeria to meet the needs of taking cohorts of people through a Staged Change on different social platforms such as market places, schools, churches, etc.

CHAPTER 4
4-STAGE INTUITIVE MODEL
OF BEHAVIOUR CHANGE

INTRODUCTION

It is against the background of the interaction of the level of personal freedom and initiative and the cultural hold on behaviour that the intuitive 4-Stage model of behaviour change (hence forth referred to as the 4-stage framework) was tailored to the Yoruba world view and operations of personal choices. Each of the stages is now briefly discussed to show the operational implications and the contribution each stage makes to subsequent stages. Each stage is cast in the form of providing answers to the health concern.

THE INTUITIVE MODEL PRESENTED AND EXPLAINED

In order to facilitate the presentation of materials from different projects in subsequent chapters, it is advisable that we begin with the components of the derived 4-stage framework in its full developed form. That way, it will be easier to appreciate how each of the projects took the starting intuition a step further from the proof of concept to the validation of the framework.

There are four essential stages, each of which has some relationships to existing theories but whose focus is the unique context of traditional (non-modern) societies of which the Yoruba is but one of many in the country.

Stage 1: Is there any danger? (Confront)

In the absence of a scientific body of knowledge of what constitutes health hazards, the emergence of an unknown syndrome and its recognition as a source of health concern to individuals or groups are two different things. Pre-contemplation is largely ruled out when the emergence is gradual and has disseminated into the population before its official recognition as a public health problem. In such circumstances, the recognition of the health hazard is likely to be based on confronting the public with the hazard or danger. Consequently, the first stage of health behaviour modification for the Yoruba is to ask: "Nje ewu mbe?" Is there any danger?

The confrontation arises from the differences between traditional notions of danger and their origins and the modern notions offered them by the public health officials and their agents. After the first documentation of HIV infection in Nigeria in 1986, the prevalence rate increased fairly rapidly from 1.8% in 1991 to 5.8% in 2001. Subsequently, there was an irregular pattern of short term declines and increases in prevalence rates which stood at 4.4% in 2008 and down to 3.4% in the 2012 survey of

National HIV/AIDS and Reproductive Health Survey-Plus (NARHS Plus). The recognition of the present and imminent danger from HIV took various elements into consideration. The proportion of population exposed to media on HIV prevention increased, the proportion of population showing up with AIDS also increased. The personal knowledge of persons who have been infected or died from AIDS also increased (Federal Ministry of Health, 1991, 1999, 2001, 2003, 2005, 2008, 2010, 2012).

In dealing with target audiences, individuals or groups, therefore, the initial purpose is to make sure that the confrontation of the reality of the epidemic takes place. This may require a number of measures. Within the limitations of their own world view or non-scientific background, the basic features of the epidemic must be presented in terms which they can understand. The causes and effects well established and proven must be explained to them irrespective of whether those causes and effects are represented in their lives or not. The range of options in the transmission and the prevention must also be presented. Equally useful is any multimedia material with which some of the co-factors of infection can be explained. A central one is the link between other STDs and the elevated risk of HIV infection. In this connection, the gross anatomical details of advanced untreated cases of cancroids as an example of the devastation that STDs can cause, as well as the facilitation of infection which conditions create, are powerful tools of confronting the audience with the substantial dangers that HIV infection pose. Providing information, either as testimonies or case studies, of the impact that HIV infection and AIDS can cause in the domestic economy can also help make the secondary impact of the epidemic appreciated as a significant undesirable outcome of infection. In a study conducted by this author on the household effects of HIV/AIDS in Uganda (Adeokun, 1996), a strong relationship was shown between the adoption of HIV prevention strategies and the observable consequences of high HIV prevalence in an area. In some local communities, nearly half of the households had lost members or have people suffering from HIV/AIDS. In effect, what people are going through has a greater impact on their behaviour than what they might be experiencing later.

The choice of the materials that will cover all these issues raised remains the same for all audiences but the presentation style will depend on the socio-economic level and familiarity with different medium in the population. While the educated audience may make their own visual observations, the illiterate and unsophisticated audience may require a running commentary (Bankole, 1982). By the same token, the demonstration of prophylactic practices may be more explicit with the illiterate audience than with the educated or sophisticated one.

At this stage of confrontation, the presentation is an objective one aimed at assisting the audience to reach the conclusion that, irrespective of their own personal sexual behaviour or other HIV infection risks, the epidemic is a significant public health hazard deserving of the general public alert which the confrontation is aimed at establishing. It is when that objective reality is established that there is a present and imminent danger that the intervention can move to the second stage.

Stage 2: Am I at risk? (Conviction)

At the end of Stage 1, the confrontation may not prompt any more reaction from the audience if in their perception all the information and experiences fall out of the range of their own assessment of exposure to any risk. For conviction to occur, the audience at personal or group level must, in light of the evidence available and presented answer the question: Am I at risk?

In the theories reviewed, the emphasis is placed on behaviour change after an appreciation of vulnerability. For example, the background variables in the Theory of Reasoned Action, relate to the proposed action and takes for granted how the subject reached the conclusion that action is needed. In contrast, the Stages of Change take into account three steps leading to action, namely, the pre-contemplation, the awareness and the self re-evaluation of the current behaviour.

In the intuitive 4-Stage model, the pre-contemplation and contemplation are collapsed into the externally influenced confrontation. The self revaluation is the second stage. But for most people in pre-modern society, the limitations of knowledge base make the need for assistance or facilitation of their thought process important if this revaluation is to be competent.

There are a number of tried methods of such assisted self risk assessment that can be fitted to the conditions of a largely illiterate community. One is the role playing of some of the causes and effects presented at the awareness of danger stage. Most often, such drama sketches are devised by the audiences themselves and draw on their own life styles and experiences. They may laugh and joke in the presentation of the sketches but the process of revaluation goes on inside the individuals.

There are the anonymous responses to risk diagnosis questions – a form of sexual or risk practice history taking that can be used for risk/vulnerability assessment. This method was used quite effectively in the case of smoking and cancer association quizzes in the Readers Digest in the 1960s to 1980s. How many cigarettes do you smoke in a day? This and similar questions are asked and the reader is asked to rate their risk of cancer on a scale based on the answers they give. While the educated person can take such vulnerability tests on their own, similar tests can be administered on group basis with the responses kept private and the risk assessment scale given to the audience at the end of the test.

In this silent self examination, each individual answers five questions in their mind, hopefully, without self deception:

Figure 4.1: Schematic Presentation of the 4-Stage Intuitive Model of Behaviour Change

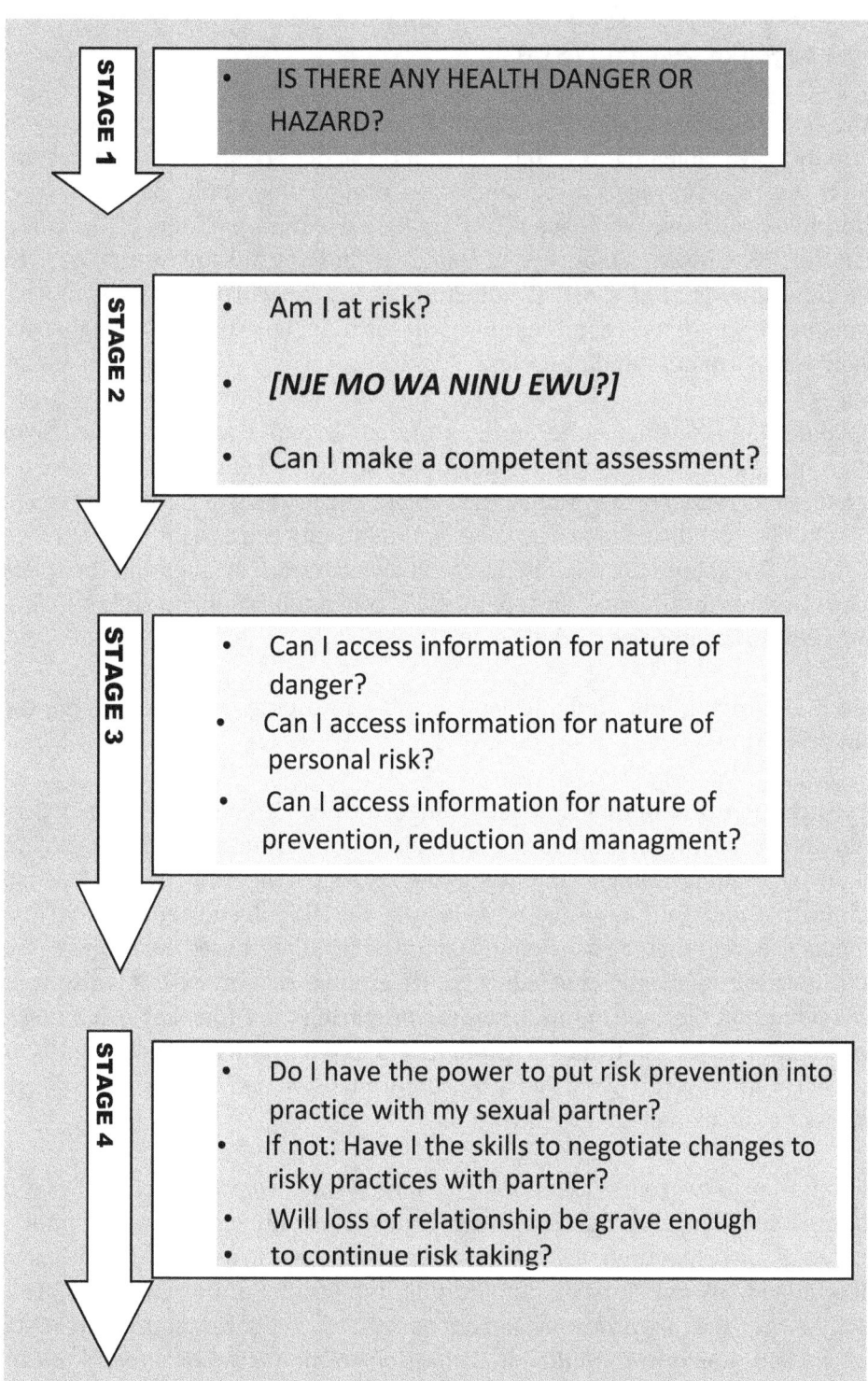

1. Are you sexually active – in/out of marriage?
2. Have you had blood transfusion recently?
3. Have you been exposed to shared non-sterile equipment?
4. Are you and your sexual partner mutually faithful?
5. Do you know your HIV STATUS?

At the end of the exercise, the facilitator can then reflect on the evidence based information available on the sexual and other practices relating to HIV infection risk and use this to encourage a discussion of the group vulnerability as well as personal vulnerability for those who have the courage to use their personal life to enrich the discussion. The obvious message, of course, is that any one answering "Yes" to first three questions is at risk of HIV infection. It is also worth emphasising that the language of discussion is a combination of the local language and use of English when it is likely to make understanding easier.

The counselling setting, either one-on-one or group counselling can form the background for risk assessment. Against the background of the awareness of danger that has been created in the mind of the subject, the probing of risk factors is a logical next step. The condition of privacy and confidentiality can assist the effectiveness of this stage. But shared forum of exchange such as drama sketches and role plays can help to reinforce the personal and confidential conviction of individuals at this stage of change within the intuitive model.

Stage 3: Acquiring knowledge, resources for reducing risk or avoiding danger (Conversion)

Once conviction of vulnerability is established, the push to action in traditional society is the "supply" of information on the knowledge and resources (including strategies) needed for avoiding, reducing or eliminating the risk of the danger of, in this instance, HIV infection, and if already infected, managing the HIV infection and its aftermath. [It becomes apparent that the conviction stage is not rigidly focused on negative issues of risk of infection but diagnosis of behaviour that reduce risks as well. It is also apparent at this point that the confrontation stage is preparing the audience for interest in the determination of infection and its management as well. Consequently, the HIV basics which form the take off event must be comprehensive and touch on the prognosis, progression and management of infection.]

The limitation of awareness creation based largely on a programme of IEC distribution is that the knowledge, resources and strategies for avoiding or managing infection is "broadcast" or distributed without discriminating between the stages of change at which individuals are situated. In addition, the variety of IEC materials are made available when they are produced and not necessarily in phases tailored to the stage of change. Consequently, the individual reaction to the materials depend upon their familiarity with the clear and imminent danger posed by the epidemic, their sense of significant vulnerability or an attitude of total indifference to the epidemic or to the topic the IEC is dealing with.

Within the 4-Stage intuitive model, however, the orderly presentation of IEC material in a way that serves to reinforce the stage of confrontation, conviction of vulnerability and conversion to taking action makes the reception and favourable consideration of the materials much more predictable than if IEC material is distributed outside of the framework of the model. For example, IEC material indicating places where HIV test can be taken can suddenly play a vital role in the prompt or cue to action for those who have been primed for the decision to test. The material will be less effective/meaningful to those for whom such information is just as input into general awareness creation. Similarly, condom negotiation exercises and training among those target groups who have been processed through staged change take on greater significance than if they are placed within the context of a broad awareness programme.

The ultimate aim of Stage 3 is that the subject be empowered to have the confidence to put their conviction into action. The more thoroughly they are equipped with the information, resources and strategies with which to cope with navigating the prevention, detection and management of infection the better their chances of moving to Stage 4. In effect, Stage 3 has the echoes of the "prompt to health action" of the HBM and the "self liberation" in the Stages of Change in the review above.

Stage 4: Acquiring the power/motivation to put knowledge to practice through negotiation, access to services and moral stamina to persevere in behaviour change without relapsing (Commitment)

In the theories and models reviewed earlier, the dominant ethos is that of the self contained individual who takes responsibility for their action within the confines of their perceptions and attitudes. The influence of relevant others is often peripheral to the formation of attitude to behaviour and any resistance to change on the ground of others' views is self imposed. In non modern societies, the conversion may still not translate to action because the subject lacks the authority to put that conversion into the practice of new patterns of behaviour.

A case in point is the resistance of male sexual partners to the uptake of female condoms when they were introduced into family planning clinics in Oyo and Lagos States in the years 1999 to 2002 (Adeokun et al., 2002). Since the dominant element in changing sexual behaviour for HIV prevention revolves around barrier method use, the direct power play involving the subject and relevant others goes beyond attitudes and perceptions and requires the empowerment to negotiate the new behaviour if need be. Although the motivation to action is invoked in the HBM, its application still places the emphasis on the self actualization of the subject rather than on the "resistance of relevant others". This omission is not present in marketing research where the influence of relevant others on marketing choices is fully articulated in Individual Choice Models.

In the 4-Stage intuitive model, the processes of vulnerability assessment and the provision of necessary resources for taking action prepare the subject for major conflicts within themselves and with relevant others which must be resolved if the final commitment of Stage 4 is to take place. This role of relevant others was touched upon in chapter 1 on what habits are and how they can be changed. In addition, attention will again return to the role that others actively rather than passively play in the realisation of behaviour change.

In considering the role of relevant others in decision making, the emphasis changes from what will others think to the real objection of those others to the line of action necessary for self preservation. In traditional society the objections can lead to further weakening of the position of the subject such as is the case when men decide that the proposal of condom use is evidence of their wife's infidelity or evidence of challenge to their marital authority. In effect, the Stage 4 in the intuitive model places the emphasis on the empowerment of the subject – most often women – who need to be able to overcome such sexual partner objection if they are to effect commitment to their proposed health action.

The actualization of Stage 4 in behaviour change communication requires that the educator or facilitator be familiar with the prevailing power relations and be able to identify point of countering the status quo. For this to be effective, the position of weakness, the costs of confronting the objections, the strategies for converting the opposition to one's views and the motivation of opposition to join the new viewpoint must all be taken into account and addressed in the behaviour change communication at this final stage of the model.

The components of Stage 4 intervention must include some of these elements:

- Negotiation skills to overcome unequal power relations – including condom use
- Access to services for prevention, testing, care and support in such a way as to allow independent line of action
- Moral stamina to persevere in the path of survival and resist temptation to revert to old habits
- Constant review of progress through periodic HIV testing and prompt treatment of other sexually transmitted infections
- Helping the relevant others to experience or share in the behaviour change process based on the 4 stages through which the subject has passed.

The nearest framework that comes to mind in handling this realignment of authority within the dyadic sexual setting is that of Organisation Control (OC) in which resistance to change can only be on the resolution of the opposing forces. According to OC the Force-Field Analysis can be employed to implement change in an organisation.

As a first step in OC, the Force Field is "un-frozen". Next the driving forces for change must be enhanced and the restraining forces retarded. Thereafter when new equilibrium is attained the Force Field must then be refrozen.

In its application to the resolution of the conflict of interests between sexual partners in the process of behaviour change, the unfreezing of the status quo in their power relations is the first step. For this to happen, the partner has to be processed through the stages of change, either by their involvement in the initial intervention or in a secondary intervention which may be carried out at the level of couple counseling at the clinic level. There are, however, some women who are relatively empowered enough to take on the responsibility of processing their partners through stages of change.

A major tool in the unfreezing of the sexual relations is to assist the partner in vulnerability assessment so that they see any concessions in sexual matters not as a favour to their partner but a self preservation strategy in the context of the HIV/AIDS epidemic. Consequently the main driving force for change in male partners is the realization that the risks of HIV infection through unprotected sex are high enough to make the adoption of barrier methods of contraception a worthwhile move.

To help the partner cope with the major restraining factor, that using a condom is not as enjoyable as without, the negative issue that not using the condom carries significant risks can affect attitude of the partner. The possibility that the use of the condom also removes anxiety about the sexual health of partners can effect such change in attitude. Once the notion of changing safe sex practices has been accepted and put to test under conditions which both parties consider as satisfactory, the new equilibrium in their relations can then be created and consolidated and re-frozen.

MATERIALS AND METHODS FOR IMPLEMENTATION OF EACH STAGE

The real test of the 4-Stage Change Model lies in finding, devising and presenting the materials and methods that will lead the target group to reach the appropriate stage-change answers to the questions posed. Such materials include audio visual materials, drama sketches developed by the group, pedagogic material passing on information from a wider cycle of local, national and international information on the epidemic.

The methodologies for the presentation of materials must be suited to the socio economic background of the group so that the level of comprehension does not become an issue in arriving at decisions on stage of change.

Step 1: Is there any danger?

The initial stage of confronting the target population with the dangers posed by the epidemic requires a balancing of the elements of relieving their ignorance, fear, anxiety, comprehension of scientific information and the appreciation of public health data upon which the individual or group can begin the process of contemplation.

In previous projects, the following has been the most effective combination of materials that can get the urgency and clear and present danger of ignoring a major sexually transmitted infection such as HIV/AIDS:

(a)   Informal discussion of the group's knowledge of the causes, progress and symptoms of familiar STDs such as gonorrhoea and syphilis – this segment should help break the ice about the discussion of sexuality in general and STDs in particular. [During the protocol for the involvement of the group, the general idea that HIV prevention is the theme of interest will make this ice breaking session not as tedious as with a group not primed for the intervention.]

(b)   Exploration of individual understanding of the basic concepts about the HIV/AIDS epidemic: What the acronyms stand for, the facts and myths that they have heard about the epidemic, personal knowledge of anyone who is living with or has died of the syndrome etc. In this segment, the HIV basic information is used as an interactive material for confirming or modifying their knowledge of the epidemic.   Specifically, the information should also cover the transmission, prevention and the message that programmes of management are increasingly becoming available. At this point if the session has been well managed, the intellectual interest of the group should be piqued and they may increasingly ask questions that form the basis of going into the next segment on the danger of HIV infection or the implications of such infection in the life of the individual, the family and community at large.

(c)   After the intellectual interest, the clear and present danger posed by the epidemic require that the group be confronted with some of the more graphic information available on the interaction between other STDs and HIV and on the progression of persons from HIV infection stage to the acquisition of full blown AIDS.

Powerful as such audio-visual materials are, those that are being used are dated and require that they be updated. Professor Ransome Kuti was the Minister of Health at the time these materials were prepared. Some of the materials were also produced in East Africa at about the same time. In a few cases, the categorical statements about the syndrome and the problems with its management are now out of date. In spite of these limitations, so effective are the film clips - Silent Epidemic and the Dawn of Reality – that showing them is preferable to not offering visual materials about STDs or some visual imagery of the advanced stages of AIDS.

(d)   Some audiences are sufficiently agitated by the visual material on gross impact of STDs that they are of the view that such conditions as untreated cancroids are demonstrably more devastating than the slow paced HIV infection. In addition to this reaction to the video material, it then helps to use some public health information so that the extent of the dissemination of the HIV/AIDS epidemic in the country can form the background to Stage 2 when the issue of personal vulnerability is up for discussion. The most salient issues about the national epidemic which are also relatively easy to communicate to an illiterate audience are as follows:

- Prevalence of HIV among Adults in Nigeria Increased from 1.8% in 1991 to 5.8% in 2001 and 5.1% in 2003 and stands at 4.4% in 2005; this needs to be updated to te latest data of 2010.
- Large State to State differences which in 2001 ranged from 1.8% (Jigawa State) to 13.5% (Benue State) and in 2003 from 1.2% (Osun State) to 12% (Akwa Ibom State). Expressed as proportions, the prevalence rates make sense irrespective of educational background.
- Large country to country differences which ranges from 1 in 5 adults (20%) to 1 in 3 adults (33%) infected (in South Africa, Zimbabwe, Botswana etc.)
- The rising proportion of deaths due to AIDS in Nigeria from 1990 when AIDS accounted for 10% of all deaths to 2005 when AIDS accounted for over 50% of all deaths (we need updated data; sources of data should be acknowledged
- The vulnerability of sexually active young people in all countries and the impact on their burden of diseases and deaths: Young people between the age of 15 and 34 have HIV prevalence rates that are twice the national infection rates and they carry a higher likelihood of death from AIDS than other age groups.

(e)   Illustration of Sexual Behaviour of Youths: from Oyo State Senior Secondary School Classes (2003) Survey evidence can be presented in aggregated form without compromising the confidentiality of individual responses:

- 45.9% reported having a boy/girl friend.
- 20% have had sexual intercourse.
- Over 40% had their first sex between age 12 and 16
- Of the sexually active in previous 3 months, 72% had more than one sexual partner.
- Less than 10% have ever used a contraceptive before most often the male condom

At the end of the segments, the group discusses the issues raised, ask questions for clarification and then confront the question posed in the form of [do we have reasons to be concerned or worried or fear the prospect of HIV epidemic. Does the epidemic pose a clear and present danger to the individual, community and the larger society? The ambiguity surrounding the various concepts of danger, hazard and so on is resolved in the local language by the phrase: Njẹ Ewu Mbê? [See discussion on the fear of death and other phenomenon in Yoruba psyche.]] Usually, the conclusion is reached in loud acclamation that indeed, the HIV/AIDS epidemic is a clear and present danger to society: Ewu Mbê!

Step 2: Am I in danger or at HIV risk?

The speed with which this second stage is embarked upon depends on the agenda for the training intervention. But conceptually, a period of reflection after the events of confrontation in Stage 1 is advisable. In any case, the materials to be absorbed in Stage 1 can take more than a day depending on the amount of excitement and insight generated among the participants. In general, the quality of the facilitation is the prime factor in that excitement and insight. At times, the exposure to media information and familiarity with HIV basics may make the progress towards rounding up Stage 1 on the very first day of training possible.

In preparation for the vulnerability assessment, the HIV basics need to be reviewed with particular attention to the mechanisms of infection in lay terms. The reason why an open sore on the genitalia facilitates the entry of HIV is within the grasp of the least educated audiences provided the facilitator is up to the task of discussing issues of sexuality without trivialising the discussion and without allowing the discussion to degenerate into chaos.

The segment on self examination of risks of HIV infection is usually relatively short. Each individual is advised to give confidential answers to five questions (in their mind) without voicing their responses and without self deception! At the end of the reading out of the questions, with pauses in between for reflection, the scoring system is explained and the relative risks of infection attached to the scores are also discussed. Finally, the link between each of the queries and the probability of HIV infection can then be openly discussed. This openness tends to encourage the sharing of experiences and information and their knowledge of cases of HIV infection and life style issues.

1. Are you sexually active – in/out of marriage?
2. Have you had blood transfusion recently?
3. Have you been exposed to shared non-sterile equipment?
4. Are you and your sexual partner mutually faithful?
5. Do you know your HIV STATUS?

Here are a few of the issues raised in the discussion of each of the filter questions:
Being sexually active

The fact of sexual activity is a precondition to exposure to STDs. Such exposure is independent of the marital status but dependent on the nature of the sexual network into which the sexual activity integrates the individual. The fidelity of sexual partners who are uninfected or the consistent use of barrier methods are two ways of reducing or eliminating the risk of STDs. Needless to say, the verification of the STD status of the partners is a precondition for the degree of confidence they can have in their protection from infection.

Discussion of these issues linkages raise the wider issues of the high level of promiscuity in society and the difficulty of introducing condom use into marital unions without raising the suspicion of one of the partners or into relationships in which sexual activity is aimed at procreation. The point should also be stressed that the issue of sex is listed first because of its importance in HIV transmission; a large majority of Nigerians become infected through sex.

Recent blood transfusion

Although the use of blood transfusion among the general population is not well documented, there is a clear difference in the frequency of transfusion between males and females. During the reproductive years and especially during delivery, the use of blood transfusion to make up for some of the nutritional and other deficiencies in pregnancy is quite common. Explaining that the danger posed by unscreened blood is much higher due to the volume of transfused material than for other sources of infection is important so as to reduce the burden of infection among mothers and their infants on this account.

In general, the differential in frequency of transfusion should emerge if put into an open vote. The focus on recent transfusion should also be clarified in terms of the improvements in blood safety in the public health system. The relatively poorer blood screening services in the private sector are potential source of worry in public health. It should be stressed that people should receive care from government registered facilities; clients also have the right to ask their health providers if the blood to be transfused has been screened

Sharing non-sterile equipment

In the same way as with blood transfusion, the extent of sharing of non-sterile equipment within or outside the health service system is not easily documented. But there is evidence that this contributes to the transmission of HIV from person to person. The direction of exchange is either from patients to health carers of vice versa. Outside of the health care system, there is also significant use of non-sterile equipment in the practice of various skin piercing activities including circumcision, scarification and tattooing. In parts of Nigeria the practice of circumcision either in infancy or later in life is so pervasive that it constitutes a major threat in the spread of HIV from clients of circumcision. The procedures used in the traditional system often involve the cutting of a large number of clients in a session. This arrangement further increases the risk of exchange of HIV infected blood from one client to a number of others.

In recent times, the patronage of pedicurists and other beauticians create settings in which infected body fluid exchanges are possible. The need for awareness creation about these risks arise from the innocuous nature of the procedures including the cutting of toe and finger nails in market and other locations, the scraping of hair from the head and the use of sharp tools in hair dressing and barbing saloons. Most clients take these procedures for granted and are usually appalled when the risks are brought to their attention. [This accounts for the frequent reporting of avoidance of sharing non-sterile sharp object as the HIV prevention changes people have made after an intervention.

Assurance of sexual partner mutual faithfulness

In spite of the simple logic of HIV prevention based on mutual monogamy between two HIV uninfected persons [and even among HIV infected and discordant couples], one of the most pervasive risks in sexual transmission of HIV is the extent to which people are unfaithful in their sexual lives either because they have many partners as a life style or because their partners also have other partners. In addition, sexually active persons use different strategies to discriminate in their prophylactic practices. As discussed in Chapter 3, even those who are commercial sex workers make distinctions in their use of condom.

Apart from promiscuity and commercial sex work, there is a dominant ethos of male infidelity that manifests in the survey evidence discussed also in Chapter 3, in which apparently, two-thirds of married women are either certain their husbands have other sexual partners or are not sure that they do not have. This leaves a third of women who by their own account have mutually faithful partners. The possibility of the further reduction of this group through the surreptitious infidelity of their husbands cannot be ruled out.

Knowing one's HIV status
In any epidemic, a major risk is ignorance of the infective state in which one is in. In the case of HIV/AIDS, such ignorance is potentially deadly. Because of the varied history of the syndrome from person to person and from circumstance of infection to another, knowing one's HIV status becomes a vital survival strategy. Drawing attention to the gap in their knowledge can act as an important prompt or cue to take the HIV test during, or soon after the intervention on vulnerability assessment.

The attraction of knowing the HIV status after prevention interventions is that the knowledge can help shape their future sexual practices even if they are not already infected and if they are infected shape their health care seeking behaviour relating to the management of the infection. As the provision of anti-retroviral therapy increases and HIV infected individuals are known to be staying healthy and even those at the advanced stages of AIDS are shown to recover, in some cases, quite dramatically from their symptoms, the benefit of early diagnosis and treatment is becoming more comprehensible to the general population and can be communicated effectively within HIV prevention interventions.

Plenary discussion of the Segment Question: Am I at risk?

The purpose of the plenary is to give an opportunity for the outpouring of feelings that get pent up during the discussion of the risk factors. Another purpose is to allow for the inevitable clarification of mistaken notions and myths that people hold about the causation of HIV infection.

In the end, the greatest benefit of the segment on risk assessment is that it should reveal the inclusive nature of some of the risks so that no one feels complacent about their exception from the risks on account of their previous perceptions of safety.

Step 3: Acquisition of knowledge, resources and motivation

Concept clarification

Knowledge comes in media, formal communication in training sessions, public enlightenment campaigns, health talks and one-on-one counselling settings. Informal communication takes place in various settings and is largely based on interpersonal exchanges of unstructured information.

Resources include access to prevention, testing, care and support information. Motivation is the outcome of "Conversion" to the new values and the recognition of the benefits of the new values. It implies a cost benefit analysis of not changing habits.

Knowledge acquisition
In general, the exposure to non-specific general information about the HIV epidemic on radio or in the mass media is the earliest entry point into the awareness, prevention and management of infection. Such exposure is irrespective of the recognition of personal vulnerability of full appreciation of the messages passed on in the media [an area for further research].

Whatever the source of information, progress to taking action is not linear and the process of contemplation, reception of cues or recognition of personal vulnerability may be hindered because the broadcast system of information sharing states general principles and not confront the audience. At the point of saturation, people may listen to the message but not hear them. That deadening of the audience's reception of information is the most counterproductive of this approach to behaviour change.

Resources for action [include access to prevention, testing, care and support information]
This is similar to Lewin's position that the adoption of new behaviour often requires

new skills, knowledge and social support to help make the change and sustain it over time. However, those resources and their mix depend upon the technological and material culture of the people and their cultural institutions.

One outcome of orderly approach to BCC is the preparing of the mind for filtering information received much more effectively than if the mind was unprepared. The information covers all phases of action from prevention of infection, testing for infection accessing care and support. Without the awareness of the epidemic and the sense of vulnerability, the information provided in the media on HIV prevention does not arrest the attention of most audiences. Similarly the acquisition of a condom has to be a conscious pre-sexual activity decision and not after the fact. This is only possible when people are aware of the risks of unprotected sexual activity and of their own risks.

As a piece of information, a list of voluntary counselling and testing clinics may not get the attention of someone indifferent to HIV prevention but will be noticed and analysed for location and convenience by someone on the verge of taking the test.

One of the greatest frustrations reported by PLWHA is the high direct and indirect costs of access to ARV treatment. Consequently the solution of access problems can impact on the adherence and effectiveness of treatment. Left unresolved, poor access can reduce the uptake of treatment, increase the incidence of drug resistance and discourage programme planners.

Even when treatment is effective, the quality of support and care that persons living with HIV/AIDS receive from relevant others including family, friends and relations and organisations can determine the quality of life that the PLWHA lead. This is the basis of the programme preference for people testing for HIV to have some other persons with whom they are prepared to share the result of their tests and upon whom they can rely for psycho-social support. In that sense the sharing of test result provides access to other resources that may not be available if no one else is aware of the HIV status of people.

Motivation to take action *[the outcome of "conversion" to the new values and the recognition of the benefits of the new values. It implies a cost benefit analysis of not changing habits]*

The motivation to take action may, on the surface, appear a generic notion that is universal: That people will not take a health action unless they think that the action will produce the expected outcome. But the assessment of action in a modern society is different from that of the traditional society. There are imperfections in the cost and benefit analysis of action. Poverty may impose restraints to action even when there are other factors motivating people towards taking action. It is in this context that the assistance given in vulnerability assessment should be extended to the assessment of the cost of not changing behaviour vis-a-vis the benefits (short and medium term) of changing behaviour.

For avoidance of doubt, the motivation to take action is primed by the awareness and vulnerability stages. The inability of the subject to take into full account all aspects of the cost benefit analysis of taking action should not then be allowed to abort the behaviour change process. This assisted cost benefit analysis becomes part of the skills and resources with which subjects should be provided.

Step 4: Acquisition of power to put knowledge to practice

In the personal control of most aspects of life and the guarantee of rights, the decision to put knowledge and resources to use rests squarely within the power of the individual. In contrast the culture of male dominance pervading most traditional societies in almost all spheres of life put the control of children, women and material resources at the disposition of males. This control is exercised at all stages of life. Males are subject to different sexual mores from those applying to females within or outside marriage. In effect, it takes more than recognition of a health hazard and of one's vulnerability and access to the resources for action to put the knowledge and resources into the practice of changed behaviour.

The literature on constraints to condom use in Nigeria repeatedly cites the opposition of males to condom use. The same male objection has also affected the promotion of female condoms into widespread use, not because the women are not aware of their prophylactic needs and of the female focus of the devise but because the male partners do not go along with their wishes. The very advantage that female condoms can be initiated and put in place by the women prior to sexual activity becomes a negative issue with males who consider that such independence of action will encourage infidelity of women, the fact that males are involved with other sexual partners notwithstanding.

In view of this disadvantaged position of females in the sexual interaction, there are a number of measures that constitute the empowerment of sexual partners if they are to be able to translate their awareness, vulnerability and knowledge base into actual practice of safe health promoting practices. These measures are:
   a. Communication and negotiation skills to overcome unequal power relations in sexual encounters with particular attention to condom use negotiation.
   b. Provision of services for prevention, testing, care and support and unfettered access to such services.
   c. Encouragement of moral stamina to persevere in the path of survival and resist temptation to revert to old habits.
   d. Opportunities for review of progress through periodic HIV testing and prompt treatment of other sexually transmitted infections so as to reinforce the new pattern of behaviour.

e. Communication and negotiation skills.

In as much as the idea of converting relevant others to one's point of view undermines the status quo, this segment of Stage 4 of the Change model is not to be taken lightly. It often calls on all the variety of skill acquisition techniques. In the preparation of the training session, pedagogic material on negotiation of safer sex, role play, unobserved practicum in the setting of their private sexual life, review of progress in periodic meetings with subjects, and revisiting the topic of negotiating skills during clinic contacts, especially among those who are concordantly, or discordantly HIV infected will be required.

The importance of the use of role play is based on the fact that for most of the participants, such role play marks a maiden exposure to the possibility of confronting and converting their sexual partners to the new framework of surviving the HIV/AIDS epidemic through the modification of entrenched sexual practices.

Another approach to enhancing the utility of the role play sessions is to encourage the participants to put up drama sketches illustrating existing practices and incorporate some of the methods of negotiation to which they have been exposed at the training. Encouraging the male participants to become involved in the process is one way of making males aware that the change in behaviour is as relevant to them as it is to the female participants. [From experience, such male involvement and the responding enthusiasm start at Stage 1 and certainly after Stage 2 when their complacency about the risk of infection is challenged with the evidence.]
Provision of services for prevention, testing, care and support and unfettered access to such services

There are situations in which the lack of services is the ultimate constraint to practising what one believes and has the power to practice. Consequently, the provision of services within the health system is central to effective behaviour change and the sustenance of the new behaviour. This integrity of the health system is crucial at every stage from HIV prevention, testing and accessing care and support.

Along with that integrity the provision of services should not be discriminatory so that people are denied access on account of their social, economic or cultural background. By the same token, services should attempt to overcome the inherent disadvantages that people may suffer from. The free provision of ARV is one such compensation for the poverty of most people in developing countries. A decentralisation of some repeated services will also reduce the indirect cost of care to people by bringing services closer to where they live.

In the absence of traditional institutions for some forms of support and the dislocation of family economy because of the opportunity cost of providing care and support, innovative ways need to be found to create the coping capacity within communities by training cadre of care givers and providing some remuneration for some care givers because of lost employment opportunities arising from the HIV infection of family members.

Encouragement of moral stamina [to persevere in the path of survival and resist temptation to revert to old habits]

In the discussion of existing theories and models, attention was drawn to the unavoidable to return to that which is habitual either because of the loss of rewards of the old behaviour. Consequently, there is a place for the provision of support to make people persevere in the new behaviour even when there are temptations and attractions and rewards for relapsing into the old patterns of behaviour. There are institutions in society which can handle this responsibility within the HIV prevention paradigm. Religious bodies are well placed to provide this moral support to their members. There are of course limitations to what such bodies will support on the basis of the extant dogma. Consequently, the Catholic Church is not going to lend its support to the use of condoms. Other churches though may see no problem to such support even if such support imply approval of actions that fall outside of their code of fidelity within marriage, avoidance of pre-marital sex and similar ones. Such support is generally given in view of the overwhelming evidence of the irregularities in people's sexual behaviour and departure from the ideals of what such sexual behaviour should morally be.

In the prevention of relapse into old habits, there is a role for the creation of some legal sanctions that will facilitate the practice of new habits. In the wisdom of hindsight, the legalization of commercial sex work in Senegal and the provision of support services to such workers allowed their health to be a major factor in keeping the spread lower than it could have been if sex work was driven underground by punitive sanctions.

Opportunities for review of progress
One major aspect of empowerment is the creation of opportunities to review progress that has been made so that any problems arising from power relations with others can be rectified. The provision of a forum where volunteers, trainees and other participants in BCC can review progress becomes a useful tool of assuring commitment to new patterns of behaviour. It also provides the occasion for updating their knowledge about all aspects of the behaviour change process.

PART II
EVOLUTION, APPLICATION
AND EVALUATION
OF THE 4-STAGE MODEL

CHAPTER 5
PROMOTING DUAL PROTECTION IN SIX IBADAN FAMILY PLANNING CLINICS

INTRODUCTION

With the establishment of the structural and conceptual links between the conventional (western) HBM and the intuitive 4-stage framework in broad theoretical outlines in Part I, attention is turned in Part II to the transformation and development of the 4-stage framework from a proof of concept on how best to effect behaviour change in a non-western society that has a number of factors that complicate the western societal assumptions upon which those models are based. The differences between those assumptions and the realities of non-western societies have been presented in those earlier chapters. It was against the background of those differences, that the validation of the intuitive model went through phases starting from the proof of concept, to the testing of the concept in relatively favourable institutional settings, followed by its application among groups of the general population, before its robustness could be assured.

Fortunately, a number of projects were conducted from 1998 to 2010 by the Association for Reproductive and Family Health (ARFH), Ibadan, Nigeria, first in collaboration with the HIV Centre for Clinical and Behavioural Studies, New York, NY 10003 between 1998 and 2002, and subsequently with the AIDS Prevention Initiative in Nigeria (APIN) between 2000 and 2010. This made possible an uninterrupted process (from the proof of the 4-stage framework, a trial of the framework among family planning clients and the scaling up of the framework that allowed an empirically verifiable process and outcomes, which made the 4-stage Intuitive Yoruba based framework worthy of dissemination in this book form. This will allow a wider application in the ongoing battle to effect HIV prevention behaviour changes in Nigeria and elsewhere in other traditional societies. It will also be relevant to tackling other health hazards such as the Ebola outbreak that made its first appearance in the West African region in March 2014. The behaviour change requirements may vary from hazard to hazard, but the principles behind the 4-stage framework remain valid nevertheless.

The best situation for such proof was to start with a soft target so that the feasibility could be established and the concept appropriately refined. Family planning clinics and their clients offered the ideal setting. Why? The clients had taken a prior decision to do something about their family formation goals by going to family planning clinics. They were on the path to behaviour change in matters relating to their reproductive health and practices. Consequently, it was apparent that the 4-stage framework was not an exact fit to their situations. However such FP clients provided an opportunity to see how the pattern of behaviour change among them fitted into the 4-stage framework.

The first of the series of studies involving the proof of concept and the emergence of the main elements of the 4-stage framework was the promotion of Dual Protection (DP) in the following six FP Clinics in Ibadan:

1. Adeoyo Maternity Hospital FP Clinic owned by the State Government
2. Jericho Nursing Home FP Clinic owned by the State Government
3. Oni Memorial Children's Hospital FP Clinic owned by the State Government
4. Planned Parenthood Federation of Nigeria FP Clinic owned by PPFN (an NGO)
5. ARFH Main Clinic owned by the Association for Reproductive and Family Health, and
6. ARFH Satellite Clinic owned by the same NGO.

Given that the clients had been made aware of the FP services or were seeking information on such services, the framework which was available to the project team to move them on to the concept of risk assessment was the Female Initiated Protection Paradigm (FIPP) (Mantell et al., 2006). In this framework, there was an emphasis on the extent to which the awareness of vulnerability formed the basis of the choices that the women made in the process of adopting the condom, especially the female one, as the basis of their DP practices.

However there was no doubt that the project was timely in the context of the emerging HIV/AIDS epidemic. In 1998 when the project was initiated with a grant from Worlds AIDS Foundation (WAF), it was apparent that the government had a false sense of security as far as the epidemic was concerned. This was because of initial slow pace of propagation HIV/AIDs and the impression that things were not going to be as bad as in the Eastern and Southern African epidemics. The whole concept of DP was being discussed but with no formal policy or active programmes. The WAF sponsored DP project was consequently a pioneering effort and an ideal situation in which to pursue the issue of how behaviour is changed in an epidemic. In the outline of the project below, the emphasis is on the design, the methods and the strategies which allowed the lessons of behaviour change to be learnt and for appropriate adjustments to be made to the implementation in order to achieve improved behaviour change outcomes.

CIRCUMSTANCE SURROUNDING THE DUAL PROTECTION PROJECT

The circumstances behind the series of HIV prevention projects of which the Promotion of Dual Protection (DP) in six Ibadan Family Planning Clinics was the first; are to be found in the evolution of HIV/AIDS epidemic in Nigeria. That is, from the first identification of the virus in Nigeria in 1986 to its rapid propagation in different parts of the country by the end of the 20th century.

In a decade and a half the virus HIV prevalence rose from zero to a range between 1 and

7 in different parts of the country. The same variation in prevalence rates also existed in Oyo State with the southern sentinel sites recording lower prevalence than the northern parts of the state. The sentinel survey data indicated that Nigeria was confronting an increasing AIDS epidemic and that the infection had achieved a broad distribution across the country. HIV prevalence increased from 1.8% in 1991 to 2.2% in 1994 to 4.5% in 1997 and nearly 6.0% in 1999. Thus, risks, susceptibility and infection had shifted from commercial sex and transport workers to the general (male and female) population. In some geographic regions and in certain sentinel populations, HIV prevalence was substantially higher than the national rate (UNFPA, 2006; Nigeria Federal Ministry of Health, 2000).

Another feature of the sentinel data on the epidemic is the age specific distribution that shows the highest HIV prevalence rates recorded for ANC women of age group 15-19 year. In the Southwest Zone, for example, the age group recorded 5% whilst the other age groups recorded 4.5%. The data reinforced the epidemiological observations from elsewhere in Africa that young people in general and ANC women in particular constitute vulnerable groups. The urban centres also stand out as associated with elevated risk of HIV infection.

The policy and programmatic response to the epidemic slowly gathered momentum. Mass media campaign about the epidemic focused on the sensational elements such as AIDS being a "killer disease", AIDS "has no cure" and on the broad message of using condoms as the means of preventing infection. Despite the high level of awareness of HIV/AIDS thus created especially in urban areas, knowledge of the ways to prevent the disease was not so widespread. Behaviour change was slow. Although the levels of ever having used a male condom for either FP or STI prevention reported by both men (37.7%) and women (20.4%) increased according to the 1999 Nigerian Demographic Health Survey (National Population Commission, 2000), the population's vulnerability to HIV/STIs remained high. Consequently, the need for prevention education and behavioural change remained massive. Judging from the dynamics of the devastating epidemic in eastern and southern Africa, it was clear that Nigeria needed to launch vigorous AIDS prevention and control measures to mitigate its impact. Inevitably, it was not enough to have population control programmes without making sexually transmitted infections part of the mix. The logical solution was to adopt the concept of dual protection (DP) within the family planning programmes so that there can be concurrent protection from pregnancy and sexually transmitted infections.

Dual protection (DP) can be achieved by using an effective contraceptive method (IUCD, Pill, or Hormonal Injections) in combination with a male or female condom (FC), or by using a male or female condom alone or backed up by the use of Emergency Contraceptive Pills (ECP) in case of condom failure. Although the promotion of the condom is an integral component of DP, DP practice can also be achieved through mutual monogamy between sexually active, non-HIV-infected partners in conjunction with repeated HIV testing and use of effective contraception. However, abstinence, or avoidance of penetrative sex, is another means of achieving dual protection.

A dual protection strategy implies:

1.   Equal attention to men, women and their disease and pregnancy prevention needs;
2.   Assisting clients in determining their actual HIV/STI risks and helping them make the best decisions with regard to dual protection;
3.   Acceptance by family planning providers of the condom as an effective method of contraception;
4.   Assuring that condoms are available, affordable and of good quality;
5.   Counseling on the importance of correct and consistent condom use.

Dual protection is particularly important for men and women who put themselves and their partners at risk because of their own high-risk sexual behaviour. It is equally essential for sexually active people in settings where the prevalence of STIs or HIV or both is high. DP is necessary for those who have an STI or are HIV positive and for their partners so as to prevent the transmission to a discordant partner. DP is also useful in avoiding re-infection after people have been treated for STIs.

From the foregoing, it is possible to see the association of the different strategies and the stages of the 4-stage framework. Strategy 1 focuses on the awareness creation stage. And Strategy 2 approximates the personal vulnerability stage of the 4-stage framework. In the case of the clients, the awareness of some family formation problems informed their patronage of the FP clinics. And their vulnerability was apparent in their adoption of FP services. Strategies 3, 4 and 5 form part of the matrix of service environment and information requirements of stage 3 of the 4-stage framework. Missing from the strategies was the neglect of the empowerment issues which was a pre-requisite for joint decision making and concurrence between sexual partners even when one partner was reluctant. This neglect turned out to be the Achilles heel of the FP based promotion of DP among female clients since the readiness to try out the Female Condom (FC) did not translate into actual use of the device due to the failure to secure the approval of their male sexual partners.

Social and economic factors in the vulnerability of Nigerian women

Nigerian women are particularly vulnerable to HIV and other STIs due to a number of social and economic factors. Multiple sexual partnerships, within and outside of marital unions, among both women and men are high. In the rural Yoruba-Ekiti community of southwest Nigeria, not far from Ibadan, 62% of the men compared to 47% of the women reported having sex outside of marriage in the previous year (Caldwell, Caldwell and Orubuloye 1992). In addition, traditional gender roles and norms make negotiation over sexual practices and barrier contraceptives method use difficult. Many women use contraceptives to prevent unintended pregnancy and do not adequately take into account, or are unaware of their partner's HIV risk behaviours and therefore do not perceive the need for disease protection (Ehrhardt and Exner, 2000; Gerrard, Gibbons, & Bushman, 1996). When risk perception is low, so is barrier method use, especially among women with regular partners.

Because of the main emphasis of FP on population control, the ideology of the FP field has been oriented towards promotion of the most effective contraceptive methods for preventing or spacing pregnancies. In practice, this has often been translated into promoting methods that are less user-dependent. Consequently, the male condom has been perceived to be less effective than hormonal methods and the IUD. However, from its review of evidence-based data, NIH/CDC Consensus Panel in 2000 concluded that the male condom was highly effective in preventing HIV infection in women and men, and gonorrhoea in men when used correctly and consistently. Recent indication that the failure rate of condom in HIV prevention can be as high as 10% (Fitch, 2001) still positions barrier methods as one of the most effective defences against the epidemic.

The result of this ideology of FP was that the most effective and frequently used contraceptive methods in Nigeria - oral contraceptives, IUDs, and hormonal injections - provide no protection whatsoever against HIV/STIs while condoms, which prevent HIV/STIs, are poorly promoted by FP providers due to their concern that they may be less effective in preventing pregnancy; and not seeing themselves as responsible for disease prevention. Even when FP providers are trained in HIV/AIDS and its prevention, studies elsewhere in Africa have indicated that FP providers do not actively integrate this information into their FP education and counselling. However, FP providers can wield important influence on clients' choice of contraceptive methods and can provide the counselling that will help promote condom use. Only about a quarter of clients received HIV/STI information at FP clinics where staff had been trained on HIV prevention in a series of situation analysis studies (Miller et. al., 1998). In addition, negative attitudes about condoms (e.g. they reduce sexual pleasure) also impede their use (Gordon, 1996).

Studies on the determinants of adoption of DP and interventions to increase DP consistently found in the U.S. that the more effective the primary contraceptive method was in preventing pregnancy, the less likely that women and their partners use or intend to use male condoms consistently (Cates & Stone, 1992; Cates, 1996; 1997; Sangi-Haghpeykar, Horth, & Poindexter, 2001). Unfortunately, the most highly effective pregnancy prevention methods – sterilization, hormonal and intrauterine devices (IUDs) – do not provide protection against STIs, including HIV infection.

Other health service delivery features in Nigeria also contributed to HIV/STI vulnerability. HIV/STI prevention, case identification and treatment were not viewed as a top priority in Nigeria's FP programmes, even in light of the HIV/AIDS pandemic. Reproductive health counselling with clients was often devoid of discussions of sex and the assessment of clients' and their partners' sexual risk behaviours. All these issues are crucial to the promotion of DP. The lack of attention to concurrent HIV prevention and reproductive goals in Nigeria is fostered by the perception that FP clients are at low risk for HIV and other STIs and further reinforced by separately designed and administered family planning, HIV and STI prevention programmes. Family planning clinics proved to be an ideal setting to promote DP. Large numbers of young women who are among those at highest risk of HIV/STIs and are gatekeepers of contraception are seen daily, and FP providers were and still are in an ideal position to counsel clients about the need for DP and to help them make an informed choice about methods.

The traditional compartmentalization of FP and HIV/STI services operationally has meant that many women in FP clinics receive contraceptive services with little or no evaluation of their needs for STI protection. This represents a missed opportunity since they serve large numbers of sexually active, childbearing-aged women who may be at risk for primary infection, and if pregnant, for secondary maternal-child transmission. Administrative separation of FP and HIV/STI services has also led to a focus on the condom as either a contraceptive or a disease prevention method, and the development of separate condom supply and distribution systems to government health facilities that provide both FP and disease prevention services. The condom has been the cornerstone of HIV/STD prevention efforts, but its use as a DP method within FP services has not been adequately promoted.

If all these shortcomings of prevailing FP ideology/services were to be corrected, repositioning the condom for DP required that family planning programmes and service providers reform their views as well as their services. The approach to DP will then be tailored to the social and community context of women and their male sexual partners. Although no one option will be suitable since all persons are not at equal risk for HIV/STIs and unintended pregnancy, in any setting in which DP is introduced, it had to be universally promoted so as to normalize the concept and diminish the stigma associated with HIV/STI services. Practical, feasible interventions that are effective for both pregnancy and disease prevention were urgently needed to stem the tide of HIV/AIDS and other STIs. This then was the challenge that the promotion of DP in six FP clinics faced between 1999 and 2000.

The choice of the FP clinic setting for the project

The first phase of the project DP promotion, based on the female and male condom began in the 6 FP clinics in Ibadan. Participatory methodology was used to develop a DP training programme focusing on how to achieve DP, barrier methods, sexual risk assessment, values clarification, and strategies for helping FP clients to negotiate DP with their partners. A two-week training of service providers in the participating FP clinics was conducted, with assessments prior to and following training, to document changes in providers' knowledge, attitudes and counselling practices. This focus on provider was necessary so as to make sure that they were ready to make the necessary changes so that their own perceptions do not get in the way of the proper counselling of clients. The prejudicial attitudes of providers had been a major influence on the uptake of FP methods (Richey, 2008; FHI, 2013)

The eight strategies adopted for the intervention were:

1. The formative research for the recruitment of FP clients into the DP programme and the mainstreaming of DP counselling in clinic operations;
2. The design of a training manual and development of IEC materials that addressed the needs of DP whilst at the same time tailoring the content to the logical developments as the clients move from each stage of the 4-stage framework;
3. The training of service provider at the clinics including those who counsel and help clients choose the strategy for their DP practices;
4. The deployment of MIS tools for capturing the data both for the national FP registers and for the specific project data needs;
5. Maintaining a strong and robust logistics system so that shortage of condoms (male and female) did not stall the project in any of the clinics.
6. Clinic intervention and Monitoring
7. The arrangement and conduct of ten (10) 2-hour BCC programmes for the clients at the clinic at which they can discuss the challenges they were facing at every stage of the behaviour change;
8. The conduct of monthly review meetings as forum for M&E with the providers away from their clinics in ARFH House; so that for the relatively short duration of the review they can focus on issues raised without distraction from their FP routines, and so that they can share their experiences on the project with their colleagues from other clinics.

A short description of each of the 8 strategies is necessary so that the concepts behind each one can be defined. The strategies were targeted at two sets of goals. The first set were those goals relating to the delivery of an integrated DP programme within the operational framework of the clinics – provider training, MIS, logistics etc. The other set was related to the social engineering of overall knowledge, attitudes, beliefs practices (KABP) change in the clients so that the adoption of DP was not placed in the narrow band of preventing STIs and unwanted pregnancy but formed part of a broad goal of adopting new safety measures for reducing the risk of HIV infection. Into the second group of strategies were the periodic contacts that project staff had with providers not only to assure that intervention standards were maintained but to involve them in the attitudinal and behavioural change needed for their own HIV risk reduction.

1. The formative research

The approach to the formative research was advised by the reality that the DP programme had to be universal in the clinic setting and could not be selectively introduced to client. It was apparent also that there were no exceptions to interest in

DP since all the FP clients were at the clinic because of some sexual activity related outcomes such as pregnancy, avoiding getting pregnant and episodes of STIs. Consequently, for the introduction of DP promotion into the clinics, a formative research phase involving the conduct of FGDs, group health talk and DP promotion with clients at clinic sessions as well as some field survey in the communities they came from were carried out and analysed and the results were shared at the group counselling sessions and used as point of departure for the mainstreaming of DP counselling in the clinic operational routines.

The prevailing family planning ethos

The common factor in the promotion of dual protection in Nigeria was that barrier methods played a supplementary role to the family planning clinic based population control programmes. The emphasis in such programmes was to get the most effective contraceptives to the largest number of women and to encourage them to stay on those methods for as long as needed to achieve optimum birth spacing. In such programmes, the IUCD offered the most attractive option and may have inadvertently been pushed by FP providers. IUCD offer long-term protection against unwanted pregnancy and any side effects arising could be dealt with by providers. The injectable contraceptives also offered a highly effective but short term alternative. All that was required was the discipline on the part of clients to call back for their next injection on two- or one monthly basis.

The dominant feature of all the family planning programmes was that the male condom was available in programmes that were targeted at women. Consequently, the provision of male condom was not considered as an essential part of birth control programmes. It was, at best, a token concession to male services and, at worst, an ad hoc or "casual" service. Most clinics kept little or no records of the condoms distributed and no personal details of those coming in for bulk purchase or for individual needs. In all of the programmes there were no female condoms. Nor were FCs available in the pharmacy or other retail outlets selling male condoms.

Needs and site assessment of clinics and selection of project clinics

Against these background a needs assessment in all the FP clinics in Ibadan belonging to State or Local Government was carried out and formed the basis of the six clinics that were selected as DP project clinics. What the needs assessment achieved was the confirmation of the focus of programmes on birth control needs. In nearly all clinics, IUCD and Injectable accounted for more than 90 percent of all contraceptives used by clients. The Pill accounted for most of the rest. Very little use of the infra-vaginal barrier methods were in use.

However the most revealing part of the needs assessment related to the work load, clinic procedures and provider practices within the clinics. Only two of the Ibadan FP clinics saw more than 20 clients a day. Another two saw between 10 and 15 clients a day. Others saw less than 10 clients a day.

Clinic procedures were very similar. A reception is provided for clients. All clients are received at a registration desk where old clients have their client records retrieved and new clients are registered. A counselling table set aside for some privacy is provided in some clinics while others have a separate room designated for the purpose. All the clinics have an examination room with varying degrees of adequacy. Most clinics had access to IEC materials and a couple of clinics had access to audio/visual equipment for screening educational films.

With regards to the providers, the needs assessment concluded that all the staff had all received sound family planning training. Some had been exposed to counselling training on such other topics as STI/HIV/AIDS. The providers were familiar with the use of the GATHER approach to counselling. Although there were posters on the wall illustrating the stages of GATHER the providers were sufficiently familiar with the stages to offer competent counselling without adhering rigidly to the formal stages.
There were a number of flip charts for FP counselling in use in the clinics. One was developed for use in the PPFN clinics nationwide and the other was developed by an NGO and for use in some of the State and Local government owned clinics. Individual counselling was the norm in all the clinics. Group counselling was used occasionally. Since the staff had not been exposed to the concept of DP, there was no counselling on this topic. However, the staff easily identified with the concept and thought it was a timely idea and expressed interest in learning more.

Given the very few clients seen in most of the clinics, record keeping appeared to be complete and monthly summaries fairly regular. Such summaries were sent to the respective supervising offices, namely, the regional PPFN office in the case of the PPFN clinic, the State Ministry of Health in case of the government owned clinics and to ARFH in case of the ARFH owned clinics.

In addition to family planning services, a number of other services were available in some of the clinics. Such services include immunization, antenatal care, delivery and post natal care. In the ARFH owned Main Clinic, pregnancy test and blood grouping were available on request. Needless to say, all clinics had referral services to State owned as well as private Laboratories for STIs including HIV/AIDS.

Factors in the selection of the 6 clinics

The selected clinics had adequate staff situation and level of staff training in basic family planning service delivery was generally good. The physical space and IEC resources were adequate. In addition, the two deciding factors on the selection of the six participating clinics were (a) that the number of clients be reasonable to begin with and offer potential for increase, and, (b) that there be no looming policy decisions that might affect the continued existence of the clinic. It was on these bases that the six participating FP clinics were selected. At needs assessment, these six clinics saw a combined total of 70 clients a day.

Observation and exit interviews

Following the completion of the site selection and general clinic assessment, a series of structured service provider-client observations and client exit interviews were conducted at the sites. Because of the prevailing client load, these observations and interviews were conducted with every client reporting over the period of three weeks. At the end of the period 176 women completed the interviews. Of this number 15.6% were new clients another 23.9% were "restart" family planning clients – clients coming for contraception after a period of laying off. The remaining 60.5% were visiting the clinic for resupply or a scheduled repeat visit.

Clients tended to be young, with over half (54%) aged less than 30 years. The mean number of children ever born was 3.7, with 73.7% of the clients having 4 or fewer children and 26.3% having five or more children. The open birth interval was at a mean of 78 months; only 14.7% had a youngest child less than one year of age.

Contrary to the literature on the limited level of spousal communications on reproductive health matters, including family planning, in Nigeria (Meekers and Oladosu, 1996), nine out of every ten of the clients said that they had discussions about family planning with their partners. Most clients stated that their partners were aware that they were using contraception.

Of the 176 clients interviewed, the breakdown of the method they had been using or had selected on that visit was as follows: 93 were IUCD users, 63 were using injectables, 9 used oral contraception, 5 used a spermicidal agent and 6 were using condoms. In effect, only 2.3% were using barrier methods. This profile is consistent with the clients' limited knowledge of the concept of dual protection. Only 8.6% had ever heard of the concept.

This pattern of low use of barrier methods, however, did not mean that the respondents were unaware of the risks they faced of contracting STIs including HIV/AIDS. Nearly all of the clients (96.5%) had heard about HIV/AIDS. Although most (77%) were able to describe how they could protect themselves, they apparently were not taking precautionary measures.

A quarter of clients felt that they were at little or no real risk if they had sex without using a condom. The majority felt that they were at a significant or high risk of infection with STIs if they had unprotected sex. The same pattern of awareness of risk for contracting HIV was reported. We believe that the low barrier method use may be due to the low association between the risk of infection and their contraceptive use. The possibility of taking a dual protection approach to resolving their contraceptive and prophylactic problems, therefore, seemed promising.

The pattern of sexual behaviour reported shows that 3.2% of the clients had multiple sexual partners in the previous three months while the proportion with multiple partners in the previous 12 months was 8.2%.

The level of satisfaction with existing services expressed by the clients was very high. Only 3% reported method and scheduling related reasons for dissatisfaction with the family planning services. This reported low level of dissatisfaction is concordant with the rapport and mutual respect between providers and clients observed by the research investigators during the preliminary site visits.

2.   The design of a training manual and development of IEC materials

Prior to the Ibadan DP promotion in FP clinics, training materials and IEC materials had been in use in similar projects in other countries and these were based on the FIPP. The focus of the materials was on how to assist the client leading through the process of DP adoption so that they become aware of their risks and acquire the knowledge and information to determine what to do about the risks. However, during the training some of the problems arising from the assumptions that militate against the relevance of prevailing model assumptions of the type that were discussed in Part I of this book were pointed out in design sessions. These shortcomings were addressed in the design of the new training manual and in the adaption and development of new IEC materials so as to facilitate service delivery on the project. In response to some of their observations, the IEC materials were designed to emphasise the cultural dimensions to which the clients will positively respond.

Meeting training goals – the FIPP based manual

The training goals required that there be a training of trainers, a modification of FIPP materials and the determination of the training procedures. The Master Trainers would, in turn, train FP providers in the participating clinics.

Female Initiated Protection Paradigm (FIPP) training activities

The model adopted for promoting DP behaviour is the FIPP. The FIPP intervention maximizes the impact of FP services by making them responsive to the needs of FP clients in light of the realities of the HIV/AIDS pandemic (Mantell and Weiss, 1997). HIV/STI prevention is viewed as the desired norm for all FP clients. Consequently all clients are counselled with the FIPP. This helps to identify those who are high or low risk and assist them to take necessary action. Universal counselling also reduces stigmatization which is likely to result from selective counselling of clients.

An added innovation of the FIPP approach is that it builds upon the hierarchical concept of HIV/STI counselling developed by the New York State Department of Health (1992) by incorporating a simultaneous examination of HIV/STI and pregnancy prevention risks and prevention objectives. In this context it is easier to demonstrate that methods that are best for one set of objectives may be inadequate or inappropriate for the other.

The FIPP intervention has six interrelated components:

1. HIV/STI risk assessment which must include a discussion of past and present contraceptive practices, sexual practices of self and partner and potential impediments to barrier method use.
2. Reproductive health assessment including fertility status and intentions, a thorough pelvic examination of clients who are symptomatic or who perceive they are at risk of HIV or other STIs.
3. Individualized, interactive contraceptive education assisted with suitable DP IEC materials including flip-chars and picture oriented comic style booklets.
4. Skills-building regarding barrier contraceptive use which focuses on partner negotiation and other preventive strategies.
5. Prevention, diagnosis and treatment and/or effective referral for STIs.
6. Scheduling of follow-up visits for barrier method acceptors so that problems they are having in using the barrier methods may be discussed.

Development of appropriate IEC materials

The IEC materials developed included a flip-chart that formed the basis of systematic counselling of clients about the risk assessment, risk avoidance and the modalities for adopting DP. In a series of chapters a new client is taken through the stages of introduction to reproductive system, the various methods of family planning, a personal risk assessment in terms of sexual behaviour, an introduction to the competing needs of contraception and prevention of sexually transmitted infections and the role of barrier methods in dual protection.

Other items of the IEC package were posters on male and female involvement in the adoption of DP, hand bills explaining the use of female condom, defining the concept of DP and flyers on HIV/AIDS. All the materials are available in both English and Yoruba. One major feature of the IEC development was that it was participatory. The involvement of providers in the process during their training on DP and subsequently at regular review meetings was very fruitful. The local language for DP was coined in these interactions. "ONISE MEJI" translates into English as "doing two things at a time". This is the closest approximation of the concept of "dual" which is not easy to translate. Over the course of the project nearly a hundred thousand posters and handbills were distributed at the clinics and in public awareness raising events relating to HIV prevention and to male involvement in family planning. World AIDS Day is one such occasion when these materials are distributed.

Another challenge of the IEC was the difficulties providers had in systematically using the flip chart for counselling. Although prior to the project, they had a family planning flip chart in place, as was observed in the needs assessment, these charts were not systematically put into use. The providers tended to make summary presentations from memory and skip portions of the presentation according to their assessment of the background of the client. The providers also complained that keeping to the flip chart would make their other tasks impossible as the waiting time for clients would increase dramatically and discourage patronage.

Monitoring assessment concluded that whilst the time factor was indeed a valid issue, the providers needed to master the logic of the sections of the flip chart better so that they could use the flip chart much more confidently and in less time than would be required if their presentation was clumsy. An update training session focused on the different segments that were basic for new clients and those which could be glossed over in contacts with old clients.

In the end it was obvious that although the clinics had long opening hours, the client flow was packed into a few hours. Consequently, even Adeoyo Hospital, with a team of five providers in place during clinic hours, had difficulty with keeping up with the counselling and clinical services to their clients. Part of the problem is with the workload generated by the flow of clients on IUCD. With nearly 60 percent of clients on IUCD the need for insertions, inspections and occasional removals form the bulk of daily activities.

3. The training of service provider

DP programme adaptation workshop for family planning programme managers
The materials which were available for FIPP counselling had been developed for South Africa and some social and cultural contexts had to be modified so that it could be suitable for conditions in Nigeria. For this purpose all investigators and ARFH's training team reviewed the content of the original manual and selected the modules considered appropriate to the Nigerian setting. The modules formed the basis of the formal training of the DP Programme Adaption Workshop for Family Planning Managers. The output of this workshop was a draft manual and an agenda for the two consecutive DP training workshops for service providers conducted between March 4 and May 10, 1999.

One advantage of this collaboration between Programme Managers and the Investigators was that it resulted in the development of a strategy to ensure that client services were sustained while staff participated in the DP training workshop. Apart from avoiding a decline in client services if all staff were to participate in the workshop at the same time, a plan for staff deployment that allowed for maintenance of client visits and the quality of care at the normal level throughout the first service provider training was devised. Consequently, two consecutive DP training workshops were conducted.

Twenty five participants (21 women and 4 men) attended the first DP providers' training workshop. The workshop itself generated considerable interest in the concept of DP in the family planning community in Ibadan -- to the extent that some participants had to be included from non project sites because of the eagerness of the managers to equip their staff with the knowledge of DP education and counselling.

The course content addressed: Challenge of STIS/HIV/AIDS Prevention, Counselling of FP Clients on Prevention of Unwanted Pregnancy and Sexually Transmitted Infections including AIDS, the Correct Use of Barrier Methods of Contraception, Overview of Dual Protection, Cultural and Gender Issues in Reproductive Health, Condom use and Communication Skills, HIV Counselling and Communication Skills, and Dual Protection Counselling. The use of appropriate language to counsel clients on how to negotiate with their partners for safer sex was emphasized. Small group exercises, role plays and group discussions were used to sensitize participants and create a positive attitude for Dual Protection Counselling. The participants had 2 days of practicum experience in the clinic sites. This allowed them to practice their newly acquired education and counselling skills under the supervision of the facilitators. Based on their experiences in the clinics, participants developed appropriate IEC materials in the form of jingles, flip charts, brochure, handbills and posters which could be used for their different sites. The closing session for the training took the form of a stakeholders' sensitization seminar on the importance of Dual Protection. Approximately 150 persons attended. The workshop participants were awarded certificates for a successful completion of the 10-day workshop. They were also provided with the MIS forms which were designed for the additional record keeping needs of DP.

In the second DP training workshop eighteen participants (15 women and 3 men) from DP sites and two non-DP clinics participated. The two sessions achieved the project objective of improving FP providers' performance by strengthening their skills in HIV/STI risk assessment and sexual history-taking with clients, and in developing more positive attitudes about DP. However, in contrast to the information from the exit interviews, the providers tended to underestimate their clients' risk of infection from HIV and other STIs. And they were mistaken in their perception that their clients felt that they were at low risk. It was however expected that as they implement their new DP education and counselling skills and make systematic risk assessments of their clients in the coming months and years, the service providers will appreciate their clients' level of anxiety and readiness to take the needed protection to prevent HIV and other STIs.

4.   The deployment of MIS tools and the challenges faced

The most frequently overlooked aspect of service delivery in the Nigerian health sector is the quality of the records kept and the proper processing and analysis of those records to form the basis of management and policy decisions. But with the advent of the HIV/AIDS epidemic and the sustained flow of resources into implementation and monitoring of the HIV prevention programmes, greater attention was paid to the need to maintain robust Management Information System. On this project the goal of being able to track the behaviour change in knowledge, attitude, behaviour and practices required that the MIS and its upkeep at each of the clinic be very robust and that problems be picked up at monthly provider review meetings before a substantial gap in the system was created.

The impact of the DP introduction on the services, providers and clients was sufficiently disruptive of the prevailing routine of most clinics that it was necessary during the project implementation to keep in regular contact with the providers as well as the clients. Monthly review meetings with providers allowed the monitoring of service delivery as well as the maintenance of attitudinal and behavioural changes that providers made in response to the take-off training and to the challenges of the new procedures. One aspect of procedures that raised issues was the overload which the MIS tools created for the providers to the extent that they were sure it lowered their productivity on the service delivery aspect.

The challenge of the MIS development on the project was to find a suitable way of documenting barrier methods (male and female condoms) at the six clinics. The first problem was that three of the six clinics belong to government and had an MIS in place which was significantly different from the MIS system operating in the other three clinics belonging to two different non-governmental organisations (Planned Parenthood Federation of Nigeria and ARFH). The second problem was that prior to the project details of clients asking for male condom was not recorded in any of the clinics. The term "casual" was assigned to the transactions on the records with no information on the people seeking male condom.

Thirdly, the clinics did not carry any female condoms and did not have any space on their records for the commodity. The male condom accounted for just over two percent of all client visits. Supply of male condoms was often irregular and the limited amount of sales involved meant that keeping accurate records on the commodity was not considered a priority.

In effect, the MIS developed for the DP had to solve a number of problems. It had to provide for the recording of consistent counselling of all clients, both old/continuing clients as well as those who were attending the clinics for the first time. On the other hand, the MIS had to make provision for the decisions clients take to accept or not accept to adopt DP. It was equally important that the use of barrier methods alone or in combination with an existing family planning method be distinguished in the records. The MIS also had to form the basis of recruiting the panel of acceptors and non-acceptors so that the follow up surveys could be adequately managed.

In the end the resolution of all the problems was in stages. In discussions with the providers a decision was made to produce a separate register for DP on which the basic information required for the monitoring of the project could be kept. A first design went into operation for about four months (September to December, 1999). Each client had to be entered in duplicate on the forms. The project staff would at the end of the month collate copies of the forms and analyse the information for service statistics. The clinic kept the other copy.

It became apparent when the DP registers were compared to the regular clinic registers that the additional duty of completing the DP register was onerous and that some clients did not get recorded. In subsequent discussions of the situation at the monthly review meetings, it emerged that the DP forms were not easy to combine with the peak demand of the clinic. The forms were seen as being graphically complicated even though the information sought was straightforward.

In response to the comments on the DP forms, a new DP register was put in place in December 1999. In addition it was suggested that one assistant will be designated to assist providers in completing the DP register. The inconsistencies between the regular register and the DP register reduced dramatically as a result of these operational changes.

5.   Maintaining a strong and robust logistics system

It was important that supply of condoms (male and female) be regular so that the project was not stalled in any of the clinics. The prevailing social marketing of male condom took care of the supply of that commodity. However, in the case of female condoms (FC) the product fully relied on project sources for the duration of the project. The issue of the high price of FC in a few outlets meant that the project could be jeopardized if clients were left to their own devices in the sourcing of the FC. In addition, it was felt that it was not culturally advisable to give out the project FC for free since such a procedure could devalue the product among the clients. Apart from the supply of condoms, attention was paid to the regular availability of consumables including gloves, MIS materials such as the register, the referral forms and so on.

6.   Clinic intervention and monitoring

The basic intervention on the project required that every client at the participating clinics be given full counselling on DP using as a guide the flip-chart produced for the purpose. Such systematic counselling and service delivery of DP should become an integral part of the clinic routine. Monitoring activities were aimed at achieving these two goals.

Giving every client DP counselling and keeping records

When the training of providers was completed in April 1999, they embarked on DP counselling and service delivery in the clinics. Their first task was to expose every family planning client to the concept of dual protection and assist them in making informed choices about adopting barrier methods with or without the use of other methods of contraception. In performing this task they were supplied with IEC materials and an elaborate flip chart. It was emphasised in the training of the providers that the precondition of HIV prevention was that providers, clients and individuals become aware of the risks they face, make an assessment of the extent of their exposure to infection and make a resolve to avoid infection. It was stressed that the consistency of counselling was essential if the project was to become an integral part of family planning programmes that were responsive to the challenges of HIV/AIDS. Although the providers were convinced of the need for systematic counselling, they were often constrained by the pressure on them to reduce the waiting time of clients. Those pressures affected the compliance with record keeping.

Supply and resupply of female condoms

The second task was that apart from keeping records of all DP related activities such as counselling, decisions on adopting or not adopting DP, they should supply and re-supply DP clients with barrier methods. During the first 8 months of the project intervention (May-December 1999), only supplies of male condom were available to the project. There was no funding for procurement of female condoms. The challenge in this period was that clients were given counselling on barrier methods as part of the strategy of dual protection but could not respond to the interest shown by women in the female condom. This was a frustrating time for providers, clients and research staff alike.

It was not until December 1999 that the co-investigators were able to obtain a grant of female condoms through UNAIDS. The update training on the use of the female condom and on the record keeping related to the product took place in the same month so that providers could begin full implementation of DP service delivery on January 6, 2000.

A female condom distribution policy was put in place to safeguard abuses given the wide gap between the promotional cost and the theoretical market price for female condom. Clients deciding to try out the female condom were to be given 3 free samples with advice to call back as soon as they finished the free sample. The choice of 3 was based on the need to get a quick feedback on the initial reaction to the product. On the average contact was expected to be made in about two weeks.

The pricing policy was frequently under review. The 10 US cents charged was considered by some as just right whilst others proposed a halving of the price. It was generally agreed that the free sample should not extend beyond the first contact as the evidence was there that "free" items were not as valued as those for which clients paid some fee. After a careful consideration of the economic situation it was decided that the price be maintained at 10 US cents. By October 2000, the DP programme had become sufficiently disseminated in the clinics and in the neighbouring communities to justify the ending of the free sample altogether. The evidence from the monthly statistics for the third quarter of year 2000 shows that there has not been a statistically significant drop in the purchase of female condoms.

7.   The arrangement and conduct of ten (10) 2-hour BCC programmes

In each of the clinics, arrangements were made for the conduct monthly 2-hour BCC programmes among the clients. At these sessions the clients were able to discuss the challenges they were facing at every stage of the behaviour change needed for the sustained practice of DP. The structure of those BCC programmes was tailored to the 4-stage framework. Those sessions took place at the clinics so that the disruption to the clients was limited to the time devoted to the activity.

8.   The conduct of monthly review meetings with providers as forum for M&E

In the case of the monthly review meetings with the providers, it was considered more efficient to take them away from their clinics by inviting them to ARFH House. In effect, they were able focus on issues raised without distraction from their FP routines. Coming together at review meeting allowed them to share their experiences on the project with their colleagues from other clinics.

Another input into the monthly review was the sharing of outcomes of monthly monitoring visits to clinic by project team. The monitoring visits formed the basis of assuring that standards of counselling were maintained, that records were complete and accurate, that supplies and resupplies were made on time and summary statistics were prepared at the end of each month. Unavoidably, there were external factors that occasionally affected the smooth and continuous delivery of services. Political unrest, shortages of essential commodities such as motor fuel or collapse of telephone services were some the factors affecting activities in 1999 and 2000.

The solution to the problems was to make monitoring visits as frequently as possible and to make a comprehensive assessment of the operational conditions when those visits were made. On each monitoring visit the statistics were collected, counselling procedures were observed and technical assistance was given on the spot. A monitoring report was then submitted for discussion at subsequent review meetings.
A typical meeting considered the issue of FC pricing policy and the response of clients. Repeatedly, the decision was taken to maintain the same price of US 10 cents. Other issues included how to overcome the feedback from clients that some of their male

partners did not respond favourably to the FCs. The responsibilities of providers to their clients especially in the management of STIs were also discussed at these meetings. Project reports and presentations were frequently reviewed at these meetings before they were finalized. On the basis that the token fees collected from the sales of FCs fall far short of cost recovery, a decision was made to use such fees to purchase some consumable supplies for each clinic. Items such as disinfectants and gloves for physical examination were distributed at the monthly meetings.

SIX MONTH FOLLOW UP REPORT: MAIN FINDING FROM THE 6 CLINICS

At the end of the first six months of operations at the clinics, a follow up survey to evaluate progress made was conducted. One hundred and nine clients were interviewed six months or more after they had been counselled and adopted dual protection strategy. As planned, the date of the first DP visit of those interviewed was July and August 2000. These were dates by which the full complement of IEC, male and female condom and regular monitoring of services were fully established. The registration numbers of the clients allowed the distinction between those who were old clients and those who were recent acceptors.

A comparison group of clients who were exposed to DP counselling but did not adopt was also recruited for the interviews. Only the two largest clinics were involved in the survey because they allow the timely recruitment of the needed number of interviews. In making this decision, it was noted that the two clinics account for 60 percent of all client contacts in the six participating clinics. These were the two clinics where the effort of tracing clients for follow-up was relatively rewarding. Of the 109 family planning clients, 65 or 59.7% were acceptors and 44 (40.3%) were non-acceptor comparison clients.

DP Type: Barrier methods only or in combination

The focus of analysis was on adoption of the female condom since the casual distribution of male condoms and its irregular supply made it unreliable basis of comparison. Of the 65 acceptors, only 16.2% relied on the use of female condom (FC) only, more than half (52.3%) combined FCs with IUCD whilst over a third (35.3%) combined FCs with injectable and the remaining 16.2% combined FCs with Pills.

It is apparent from this pattern of use that DP posed no direct threat to effective contraceptives being in use. On the other hand, it raised the problem of consistent use by clients if they predominantly have a backup contraceptive in place when they were not sufficiently motivated to consider the prophylactic use of the FCs. It also offers sexual partners of clients an excuse to argue that insisting on the use of the FCs amount to an accusation of their unfaithfulness or that they carry an infection that could be sexually transmitted.

Amount of female condoms distributed

An analysis of the amount of FCs distributed revealed that 57% of the acceptors continued DP beyond the free sample phase of the promotion. Below are discussions of some of the socio-demographic characteristics determining the adoption or non-adoption of DP.

Socio-demographic characteristics

Age

A third of DP acceptors were over 35 years whilst a quarter of non acceptors were in that age group. In other words, there appears to be greater attention to disease prevention among the older females and greater focus on child spacing needs among the younger women. Among the older women, the effectiveness of contraceptives was as much an issue as the prevention of infections. They were also more likely to be able to negotiate their needs with their spouses than the younger women.

Table 5.1: Age and DP decision

Age group	Acceptor	%	Control	%	Total	%
(Under 35)	(44)	66.6	(32)	74.4	(76)	69.7
(35 & over)	(22)	33.3)	(11)	25.6	(33)	30.3
TOTAL	66	100.0	43	100.0	109	100.0

Source: Project reports

Education

With regard to education, Table 5.2 below shows that although acceptors account for 60.5 percent of the respondents, the level of acceptance among the non-educated is just over 33%. Those with any education are more likely to be acceptors than those with no education. Among the educated, those with full secondary and post-secondary education are more receptive to DP than the lower education levels.

Table 5.2: Education and DP decision

Educ. Level	Acceptor	%	Control	%	Total	%
None	4	6.0	7	16.2	11	10.1
Some and full primary	22	33.3	14	32.5	36	33.0
Some and secondary	26	39.3	17	39.5	43	39.5
Post secondary	13	19.6	6	13.9	19	17.4
TOTAL	65		44	100.0	109	100.0

Source: Project reports

Method mix

The adoption of DP takes two forms. The barrier method of choice can be used on its own or in combination with an existing contraceptive. One of the issues raised by the operations research was the effect that the promotion of DP will have on switching or continuation of methods. The information from the 6-month follow up survey indicates that half the family planning clients rely on a non-barrier method of contraception while the other half combine the non-barrier and barrier methods to achieve their combined prevention of pregnancy and prevention of STIs and HIV/AIDS. For example 34/64 (53.1%) women rely on IUCD combined with condoms while 24/45 (53.3%) rely on IUCD only. 23/64 (35.9%) rely on injectable combined with condoms, while 18/45 (40%) rely on injectable only.

Number of children

The effect of family size on acceptance of DP was investigated. It would appear that there is a slight preference for DP among those with five or more children than those with fewer. This may be the composite effect of the age of the women as well as their family size. The older women with medium size families are more motivated and empowered to negotiate their prophylactic positions with their spouses or partners than are younger women.

If attention is turned to two categories of fertility, namely, those with four or fewer and those with five or more, then the differential disappears. Women with four or fewer children constitute 78.8% of acceptors and 74.5 of non acceptors.

Table 5.3: Method mix by DP status

Family planning method	No of DP acceptors	%	No of control	%	Total	%
Condoms only	3	4.7	-	-	3	2.7
Condoms + IUCD	34	53.1	-	-	34	31.2
Condom + Injectable	23	35.9	-	-	23	21.1
Condoms + Pills	4	6.2	-	-	4	3.7
IUCD only	-	-	24	53.3	24	22.0
Injectable only	-	-	18	40.0	18	16.5
Pills only	-	-	3	6.7	3	2.8
TOTAL	64	100.0	45	100.0	109	100.0

Source: Project reports

Table 5.4: Number of children by DP status

No. of children	Acceptors	%	Non Acceptors	%	Total	%
0-2	21	31.8	12	28.0	33	30.3
3-4	31	47.0	20	46.5	51	46.8
5+	14	21.2	11	25.5	25	22.9
TOTAL	66	100.0	43	100.0	109	100.0

Source: Project reports

DP Decision making process

Another major issue in DP is the ramifications of informing, educating and counselling clients on a radically different orientation to family planning. Clients are faced with the need to consider the effect of DP on their spouses participating in their family planning and being involved in the operational aspects of the research. The problem they face is primarily that created by the culture of male remoteness to family planning and reproductive health matters. This section discusses some of the findings from the project on the decision making process women go through. Initially, there is a high degree of enthusiasm among most women about the freshness of the concept of having dual protection. This enthusiasm is based on the culture of double standard which places the burden of marital fidelity on women rather than on both partners. In effect, at the end of risk assessment, most women concede that they face substantial risk of infection from the activities of their spouses. They accept that the women also have their own contributions to make to the sexual health of the couple.

This stage of risk awareness is followed by a phase of receptiveness to the nominal adoption of DP. At this stage too, they are willing to take free samples on trial.

The big let-down comes when the male partner has to be informed about the female condom or observes a renewal of interest in male condom by his partner. Most women have reservations at taking on this task as there is an implicit accusation of their partners of infidelity or being at risk of infection.

Continuation rates through complaints on record

The extent to which clients continue with services is a proxy for the level of satisfaction they have with the clinics. There are client records which allow the analysis of the frequency, purpose and treatment received on various visits. Information is available in the follow up survey for 65 DP acceptors and 44 non-DP clients.

The determinant of number of visits is the primary method and the associated complaints they generate. Those on IUCDs, Injectable and Pills have their pattern of reporting which influence return visits to the clinic. Over and above these visits are the visits related to complaints about the method of choice. Apparently, those who are combining DP with these methods have extra visits related to resupply.

A total of 1,367 visits were generated by the 107 clients over the period of a year. The highest number of visits was 10 and the least one. On average each client made 3 visits. Those clients who were DP acceptors had a mean of 14 visits compared to 10 for the non acceptors. This is a significant difference in the frequency of visits. This finding is consistent with the profile of method mix. The more than half of the clients on IUCD do not need to generate frequent visits if they do not have problems. The over 40 percent on injectable contraceptives require four to six visits a year to comply with the regime dictated by either the 2- or 3-monthly injectable. In effect, interest in DP is generating additional visits either for information or for supply of barrier methods.

Support activities for the clinics

Support activities for the clinic based interventions included the creating of awareness for DP and HIV/AIDS prevention activities in other constituencies of the society. This included the school based programmes of Life Planning Education, work with in- and out-of-school youths in promoting sexual and reproductive health. In addition, the project attempted to promote DP through peer promotion and the use of market agents in the working and trading environment of the respective groups.

DISCUSSION FOCUSING ON SIGNIFICANCE OF PARTNER CONCURRENCE WITH DP AND FC/MC

Three hypotheses informed the structure, methods and management of the project. Each of these formed the basis of the discussions of the findings in this section.

H1   **The comprehensive FIPP-based training of FP service providers in DP, sexuality and HIV/STI risk assessment will lead to increased knowledge and more favourable attitudes and practices about DP among service providers.**

The focus of the hypotheses was understandably on the attitude of the providers themselves. Their attitudes play a vital role in their communication of change and innovation to their clients. What became apparent in the process of evaluation was that the attitudes of providers also are determined by their social and demographic profile. On this front it was not possible for the project to anticipate the type of providers that would be involved.

Of the 15 providers trained and serving at one time or the other in the six clinics, a third were over 50, another third were between 40 and 49 whilst a third were under 40 years. Far more remarkable was that the staff of the three government owned clinics were on average five to ten years older than the staff of the other three private sector clinics. This pattern is consistent with the fact that the longer government employees stayed on the job the better the chances of attaining a pension right. In contrast the private sector clinics attracted the younger providers.

This profile put the government clinic providers firmly in an older generation than 70 percent of their clients. They had on the average 4 children. Their enthusiasm for DP for their clients was not in doubt but the feeling was there that only few were involved with the adoption of DP in their private lives. Although all providers were given free sample for trial during the DP training, few may have actually tried it. There is no evidence of their own participation as clients on record.

When note is taken on the tendency for the Yoruba ethnic group to defer to elders, the providers do not represent the image of the innovative or the progressive in the minds of their clients. There could be a tendency for the attitudes of the older providers to be seen as judgmental in matters of sexuality when dealing with the problems of their clients. Although there was no monitoring documentation of any bullying tactics by any provider, the timidity of the less educated clients was somewhat in the background during interactions. The exceptions to the rule are those sites where the provider is closer in age to the clients.

H2   FP clients in the clinics selected for the FIPP-based intervention will be more likely to practice dual protection than clients in the same clinics before the introduction of the intervention.

This has been the most easily demonstrated hypothesis. As far back as the baseline needs assessment, it was clear that very little use of barrier methods was taking place, at least within the clinic setting. Less than 2% of visits were related to barrier methods. Although this low level may be partly the product of non-documentation of "casual" callers for male condom, evidence from the Demographic and Health Survey lend credence to the limited use of male condoms in the large population. Consequently, the fact that nearly 60% of visits are associated with DP as a stand-alone method, or in combination with existing contraceptives is a major achievement of the project.

What has been equally remarkable is the extent to which clinic-based activities needed to be supplemented with community based activities in order to increase general awareness of the problems of HIV/STIs and of the potential of DP to reduce the spread of the epidemic. In addition, funding the DP concept has been extended to two other cities of Nigeria and the role of male involvement in DP is receiving attention in other projects. The cumulative effects of these projects owe a lot to the feasibility of the first DP promotional effort in the six Ibadan clinics.

H3   Increase in perceived risk of HIV is positively associated with barrier method use at a 6-month follow-up of DP acceptors.

There is always a difficulty in testing such a hypothesis. Since 1998, the emerging HIV/AIDS epidemic has seen some dramatic changes in the notification, public discourse and planning environment. Rates in all sentinel groups have gone up and in some by as much as 200%. The change to democratic government in the country has also facilitated the influx of donor support for awareness raising and some programming in the country. However, it is apparent that in the one issue of systematically promoting DP the Ibadan project and the extension into Lagos and Osogbo with support from the FRONTIERS project is still the only such effort in the country. Consequently, the changes in perception of risk of HIV may derive from events outside of the project. The acceptance of DP and the use of barrier methods, especially the FCs, can only be attributed to the promotional efforts on the project.

The evidence from the 6-month follow up shows also that the increases in adoption of DP derive from other factors such as age of clients, existing family size, education and the prior use of other contraceptives. To recapitulate, the older clients are keener on DP than the younger clients. The more educated are more likely to adopt DP than the less educated. And education is a powerful proxy for the knowledge base regarding the HIV/STI epidemic and may assist clients to make better risk assessment. The obverse is that the educated clients are able to better negotiate condom use with their spouses than the less educated.

In conclusion, it may have been difficult to establish the precise impact in terms of the working hypotheses but the evidence of the multiplier effects of the project are not in doubt. The evidence from the short-term impact also demonstrated the likely predictors of acceptance of DP. The information indicated areas of focus for corrective procedures so that DP can be targeted at the less educated.

10. CONCLUDING REMARKS

There have been four major lessons learnt on this project. They are based on the counselling procedure, cultural imperatives, provider attitudes and the use of regular dialogue as a monitoring tool. The other contributions of the project are reflected in the presentations and publications that are emanating from the project.

a)   The role of flip chart

DP counselling, if it is to be effective requires that every new contact be given a fair exposition of the stages from risk assessment, through acquisition of DP knowledge, to the provision of services with which to effect behaviour change. In this project, the flipchart has been a very powerful tool of assuring the uniformity of counselling. It has been well received outside Nigeria and copies have been distributed to other institutions.

b)   The power of cultural imperatives in behaviour change

Over the past three decades, the delivery of family planning services contended with the resistance of male partners to the use of condoms. In essence, services to women took that resistance for granted and provided effective contraception through reliance on highly effective contraceptives. In this project, the reliance for dual protection is on the barrier methods, both male and female condoms. Consequently, the male resistance cannot be ignored. Not only is interest in male condom vital to dual protection, the female condom requires the cooperation of male sexual partners if its use is to become agreeable and acceptable. The project revealed that the male dominance which pervades all aspects of culture hold sway in negotiating sexual practices. Changing the power balance between the sexes within sexual intercourse is crucial to adoption of dual protection. Exposing male partners to all the stages of risk assessment, increasing their knowledge of dual protection and access to dual protection services is vital to the future of the dual protection strategy for HIV prevention.

c)   Providers make a difference in project intervention

When projects are in the clinic setting, the readiness of providers to make the necessary cognitive and attitudinal changes required for adoption of new procedures is crucial to the success of project intervention. Established priorities and procedures are often ingrained in providers. Consequently, they themselves need to take on the new priorities implied in dual protection strategy for HIV prevention, if they are to be convincing promoters of behavioural change. The project revealed that this reorientation can be difficult and needs to be worked at.

d)   Regular dialogue between providers, clients and project team as monitoring tool

There are three direct stakeholders in the promotional exercise. The providers act as go-between project goals and the clients. During project intervention, the goals and objectives of the parties may be slightly different. When this happens, providing an avenue for feedback becomes a vital tool of implementation. On this project, the establishment of the monthly meetings of providers supplemented project monitoring with direct feedback at the meetings. The findings from monitoring exercises can be reviewed and the lessons put to use immediately. Similarly, the periodic advocacy events which bring clients together with providers and project staff also allow a wider dialogue between clinic clients and members of the general public.

e)   Publications

Given the pioneering nature of the project, it was important that the lessons learnt be made available to a wider audience. Consequently, an effort was made in participating in international conferences and policy forums so that the prospects for effecting sexual and reproductive health behaviour through the promotion of barrier methods could be realistically assessed.

Six presentations based on the project data sets have been developed. Collectively, these publications have identified the feasibility of integrating barrier methods and dual protection approach into regular family planning services. They have contributed to the realisation that a major obstacle to women following up their risk assessment with effective change of behaviour is the resistance of their male partners (Adeokun, et al., 2002; Mantell et al., 2000; 2000; 2000; 2001, 2001).

CONCLUSION

The project raised the feasibility of applying the 4-stage framework for behaviour change among a relatively soft target of women attending family clinics. The process revealed some of the shortcomings of the assumptions of conventional behaviour change models. Being concerned about family size and sexual health and going to family planning clinics was certainly not enough to get the women to take on the adoption of the female condom as a dual protection strategy. When it comes to sexual and domestic decision making, the male advantage prevents a smooth adoption of innovation in the sexual and reproductive health domain.

However, to make the adjustment to power relations between women and the male partners, it was observed that the male indifference to sexual and reproductive health had to be confronted by making men aware of their own vulnerability to serious STIs such as HIV. This challenge of male involvement of males in the DP adoption of their spouses is the topic of the project reported in the next chapter. It allowed the serious attempt to take on a more resistant group of people with which to test the 4-stage framework.

CHAPTER 6
INVOLVING MALE PARTNERS IN DUAL PROTECTION PRACTICES AMONG WOMEN

BACKGROUND TO MALE INVOLVEMENT

In 1998, when the promotion of dual protection started in the six Ibadan FP clinics, the very idea of dual protection was unknown in the family planning fraternity. Even the common sense meaning of dual protection as preventing unwanted pregnancy and infections of STIs was largely taken care off within barrier methods programme. That programme, as far as it related to female clients, consisted of a miniscule distribution of diaphragm and other vaginal methods. As far as male needs were concerned, the males were expected to make their own arrangements, including the occasional male walk-in for the purchase of condoms. So rare were such male clinic visits that requests for male condoms were either unrecorded or entered as "casual", with no further detail on the client.

Within the primary focus of the family planning programmes on contraception and population control, the risk of sexually transmitted infections among women was considered secondary. Most providers, prior to training on dual protection counselling and service delivery, did not pay regular attention to the infection status of their clients. The exception is that the pick-up rate for such infections was understandably higher among women on IUCDs than women on other hormonal methods. In effect, the need of male partners of FP clients was not the priority in family planning programmes.

It is against this background that a proposal to integrate a male involvement component with the promotion of DP in the six clinics was made to HORIZONS. The approval of that proposal led to the initiation of what came to be known as "Promoting Dual Protection Practices among Women and their male partners in Ibadan, Nigeria."

The overall aim of the project was to assess in the different FP settings, the feasibility of an innovative service delivery model for increasing DP behaviour among women as well as among their male partners. For the male partners, it meant creating the full range of conditions for behaviour change, that is, from awareness of the dual protection needs in their sexual and reproductive life to the acquisition of skills and resources with which to meet those needs. The objective for the continuing female clients was to increase their continuous and effectiveness of DP practice by offering continuing IEC support and problem-solving counselling. The increase in men's support for their partners' initiation and maintenance of DP behaviour was the ultimate goal.

These target population-related objectives were placed within the following specific programme objectives:

a. Enhance the FIPP based strategies employed in the earlier project among the female clients by employing the 4-stage framework as the implementing framework for the project so that the outcome in terms of turning knowledge to practice can be improved;

b. Improve FP service providers capabilities and develop more positive attitudes toward barrier contraceptive methods and DP;

c. Increase the practice of DP by clinic FP clients through education about barrier methods, including the female condom;

d. Develop and test a programme management and monitoring system to assess the degree to which DP objectives are met;

e. Develop educational, counselling and clinic based activities that will attract and encourage male partners of clinic clients and other interested males to support the practice of DP; and

f. Evaluate the extent to which the four stages of the 4-stage framework produced the BCC expected from the model.

All but the fifth of the six programme objectives were carried over from the earlier study of promoting DP primarily among female FP clients. The central effort of the expanded project was aimed at attaining a level of male friendliness that would make the FP clinics a suitable setting for males to explore their own DP practice. A related sub-objective was to encourage such attitudinal changes in male partners that will lead to a better appreciation of the joint male and female needs for DP and make males more receptive to the DP decisions of their spouses as well. The next section on methods reveals that it indeed was easier to involve male partners in attitudinal change than to make existing FP clinics dramatically more "male friendly". The reasons lie in the extent to which the reproductive health needs of the males were never, until recently, part of family planning programming in Nigeria.

METHODS

The challenges of male involvement in family planning had their origins in three target groups. The first group was made up of the providers who were trained for, and used to running female focused services. The second were the female clients who had separate encounters with providers in clinics and with their sexual partners outside the clinics. The third group was made up of male partners of clients who were aware or not aware of the family planning activities of their spouses. Such males did not need to approve or disapprove of those activities except if such activities directly interfere with their sexual pleasures or family formation intentions. Clearly, those female FP clients who involved their spouses in their birth control efforts constituted the easiest group to approach for initiating male involvement in promoting DP. In contrast, there were a proportion of clients who were clandestine family planners. Their spouses were assumed to be hostile to their intentions and required a tailored approach to their involvement. Yet a third group of males who were not partners of FP clients could have been unaware of their needs for dual protection.

In the determination of the methods of implementing the project in such a way as to assist the progress of participants along the path of the 4-stage framework, a number of activities were embarked upon with the following structures and effects:

a. Focus group discussions on various aspects of making FP clinics male relevant were organized for men, most of whom were partners of FP clients;

b. Arising from those FGDs, a series of monthly encounters between project staff and males from the neighbourhood of each clinic was initiated as a platform for encouraging the mutual support group for the attainment of the project objectives;

c. The content of those regular meetings revolved around the choice and delivery of information, education and communication that would encourage attitudinal and behaviour change in the group of regular participants who went through the behaviour change communication programme; and

d. At the end of programme implementation, various quantitative and qualitative techniques were chosen for evaluating the achievements of the programme of male partner involvement in promoting DP practices.

The content of the different components of implementation are described below with emphasis on how they foster the progress along the BCC path proposed by the 4-stage framework. But in as much as some aspects have been covered in the theoretic review of the 4-stage framework and the HBMs in Part I, such descriptions will be brief.

Recruiting male partners

In developing the strategies to reach male partners of FP clients, discussions with the providers revealed that the male interest in FP clinics was low and that male patronage was not directly linked to the activities of their spouses but to their own occasional needs for barrier methods. Since male condoms were readily available on the open market and in social marketing programmes, males used the FP clinics on the basis of how close they were to them. In contrast, some women do not necessarily use the clinics nearest their home. This was a convenience for those who wished some privacy about their FP activities. In effect, it was suggested that in the recruitment of male partners, those males who have shown some interest in casual use of male condoms and those who were easily reached from the FP clinics should not be excluded on the grounds of not being partners to a current FP client.

In the end, male partners of FP clients and other married males who were not partners were invited. The former group were invited with letters sent out through their spouses attending the clinics. The second group were invited directly by the providers on the basis of being known to them in the neighbourhood. Both categories of males did not necessary live in the neighbourhood but had their work places there. The ratio of male partners to non-partners of FP clients was about 2 to 1 at the beginning when the FGDs were being conducted.

Establishing ground rules for FGDs

The main purpose of the series of FGDs was to give the males a direct stake in the initial planning and direction of the programme. They were allowed to shape the strategies to be adopted in making their involvement meaningful and in developing solutions to problems that were anticipated at the time of FGDs. It was apparent to them that given the past history of female oriented FP services, the members of the project staff were aware of the enormous challenges to be faced.

The themes addressed in those FGDs included reproductive health needs of males, expanding scope of services in FP clinics, logistics of providing services to males and females in the same clinic when the clinics were universally female staffed, the demands of formation of a male FP support group, the preparedness of the members of the group to attend a minimum of eight monthly meetings so that the range of skills needed for absorbing the educational and behavioural change communication can be acquired.

At the end of the FGDs, a number of similar themes and ideas on strategies came from the different male groups. The most important to the format of intervention were:

a. That addressing the reproductive health needs of males was in itself worthwhile;
b. That the prospects for any radical improvement of any health service systems, under the current state of the economy, was unlikely;
c. That given the enabling environment they will make themselves available for the formation of interest groups for each of the clinic;
d. That the technical and other inputs proposed for the groups by ARFH appear adequate for now; and
e. That the groups will redirect their efforts as progress was observed.

Election of officers

Soon after the FGDs, the participants decided on their own to form themselves into informal social groups. They immediately elected "officers" who will look after their affairs, serve as contact persons for those who were more difficult to reach and act as facilitators at outreach events involving the males. This development was consistent with the traditional emphasis of having leaders to guide activities of any group. The terminologies of Chairman and Secretary were cloaks for those of them who they saw as having such leadership qualities. Age and strategic location of home or place of work played a part in the selection of Chairmen. Education and literacy was the dominant consideration in the choice of Secretaries. This very development was indicative of the seriousness they attached to the project and their readiness to make the necessary commitment to it. It did appear that the newness of the concepts of FP and DP was a major reason for the interests shown by the groups.

Regular monthly meetings and in-between – men counselling men

The purpose of the monthly meetings was to provide a regular forum for the mutual support of the members in the inculcation of dual protection concepts and values in their lives. In traditional Yoruba society, irrespective of age, the opinion of peer groups count in the individual's decisions. In the adoption of new values, looking at the response of peers is part of the behaviour change process for many (Odutolu, 2005). Consequently, the series of behaviour change communication planned with the groups stood the best chance if the group kept together and increasingly got to know one another. The front-runners encourage those lagging behind to keep up.

To keep the groups identity the issue of adding new members was addressed at the FGDs. It was explained that once the process of BCC has started, going over issues discussed earlier every time a new member joins would be disruptive of the learning process. It was decided that a once for all addition of new members at the second session was all that could be allowed. This was in cognizance of the nature of the structure of the BCC programme and the chance for the enthusiastic new member to catch up the progress made in the first session. The structure and content of that BCC is explained below.

FOUR STAGES AND OBJECTIVES OF SELF-PRESERVATION

The intuitive 4-stage framework health belief model has the following stages.
1. One cannot respond to an unknown danger. Consequently, the first step is to be made aware of the danger inherent in a given activity. The activity may be sexual, economic or trivial.
2. One would still not respond to a known danger if, in one's own evaluation, the personal risks are small or discounted. The more competently the evaluation of personal risk is conducted the more the true nature of that risk will be exposed.
3. The knowledge base for reducing risk or eliminating it completely has to be acquired.
4. Finally, knowledge does not translate to behaviour change unless there is the incentive, the resources or the power to put what is known into practice. That inability to make changes may be related to supply or demand issues. It may be the outcome of gender and other power relations. It may boil down to a matter of taste of choice.

With the model as a starting point, the opportunity in the male group programme was to tailor the intervention directly to the realization of the objectives of each stage of the model. The objectives corresponding to those stages are respectively:

1 To raise awareness of participants of the new issues in sexual and reproductive health that go beyond child spacing and welfare to the threat posed by a sexually transmitted disease to which there is currently no known cure or prevention short of use of barrier methods of contraception.

2 To assist participants, through participatory and other techniques, make a competent and informed assessment of the personal risks arising from the life choices they make, in social, economic and cultural realms.

3 To provide the range of information, education and communication materials that will allow the participants to be informed, updated and current in their avoidance or reduction of risks they face in their sexual and reproductive lives.

4 To facilitate the necessary encounter between males and their spouses in encouraging an atmosphere of dyadic decisions about their sexuality. To encourage a renegotiation of power relations that touch on risk taking within or outside marriage. To put participants in a frame of mind where the modification of behaviour is seen as a rational outcome of the knowledge base they have.

Structure of male group sessions

It was on the basis of these stages and objectives that the structure of the male group sessions were designed and modified as the situation demanded with each clinic group. In that design, a number of issues relating to the working life of the males were also taken into account. To ignore them would have been an obstacle to their full involvement in the learning and behaviour changing processes.

First, males loathe taking time off from their trades, especially if the cause is not considered worthy. Pursuing AIDS prevention and the DP strategy was initially greeted with the cynicism that not much is involved than being told to use condoms. Second, males enjoy group social activities and many belong to both secular and religious groups that provide opportunities for "going out with friends". Third, the more formal the setting the more seriously the group took the deliberations. Consequently, if the group format was to achieve its objectives, then the period of intervention needed to be long enough to encourage the bonding and mutual support that will lead to planned behaviour change.

The monthly meetings were meant to:
    a) Assure regular contacts with participants;
    b) Employ a multi-media IEC strategy so that the choice of materials could be targeted at the objectives of the different stages of the 4-stage framework;
    c) Have a minimum of eight to ten sessions of 2 hours each so as to go through

the range of behaviour changes in knowledge, attitude and practices; and

d) Acknowledge that other AIDS prevention and DP related activities will be going on in other parts of the country that will help reinforce the learning and behaviour changes going on within the groups.

In addition it was decided that after the males had completed stages 1 and 2, their spouses will be invited to participate in the other two stages so that the knowledge acquisition and the motivation towards behaviour change or modification can take place within the context of dyadic decision making of the couples. Participants were also informed of their right to drop out at any stage or to refuse to participate in any of the activities such as in the administration of questionnaires on risk assessment that was one of many activities planned.

The greatest challenge of the series was to overcome the initial awkwardness of the group participants at the predominantly female staffed and female patronage of the clinics. The capacity for male relevant services, such as screening for STIs or common ailments, had not been fully developed in any of the FP clinics. Nor were the prospects for such services high under the prevailing national policy and programming situation in the health sector.

Content of male group sessions

Stage 1: Awareness creations about the need for dual protection

The choice of IEC material was the essential input into this session. The effectiveness of the use of video materials on the ravages of untreated or poorly managed STIs and the association between STIs and HIV infections had been proved in the other AIDS prevention projects. What was required was to package the group session in such a way that the video material was placed in proper perspective and did not amount to adopting scare tactics towards raising awareness. Consequently, the first session consisted of the following elements:

1. Talk on the traditional focus of family planning on women and on population control.
2. The change in family planning emphasis in response to the epidemic of STDs and HIV/AIDS.
3. The case for male involvement. Is AIDS a problem in Nigeria? Polling of view on familiarity
   with HIV or AIDS patients.
4. Two video clips: "The Silent Epidemic (20 minutes);" "AIDS in Nigeria (40 minutes)".
5. Question and Answer and Discussions on video clips?
6. Discussion of the role of sexual networking in spread of STDs and HIV/AIDS.
7. Discussion of statements of norms and values relating to sexual networking.
8. Reaching a consensus on the threat that HIV/AIDS constitute to the individual male or female, the family and the nation.

The topics did not last more than 2 hours at each location. But, in spite of their busy schedules, the participants left the first session on a higher level of awareness of the need to pay attention to the STD/HIV/AIDS epidemic. The focus of discussion was not on the male responsibility to his wife and children or on moral aspects of sexuality, but on the individual's responsibility for self-protection and preservation so as to be able to meet those altruistic obligations to others. In other words, messages focusing on the altruistic issues in an epidemic miss the point that selfish motives or self interests underlie behaviour modification and change.

Stage 2: If AIDS is indeed real and a danger - Am I at risk?

During the second stage, a short questionnaire that documented some of the demographic, sexual and life style predictors of risk of HIV infection was prepared and administered in the course of the meeting. With the exception of a few items on current sexual behaviour, no item was obviously linked to the risk of HIV infection. These are some of the questions that each respondent answered: Do you go out with friends in the evening for an occasional drink? And do you travel away from your home base on business? In order to aid free discussion, the respondents were not expected to submit the questionnaires until the end of the session. Surrendering the questionnaire was made voluntary. No one refused to turn in the "no name, no address" questionnaire in any of the clinics.

Two of the 2-hour sessions were required for this stage. The content of the combined 4-hour sessions was as follows:
i.   A review of the impressions and lessons learnt in Stage 1;
ii.   Does HIV/AIDS constitute a potential threat?
iii.   Are you aware of cases in your neighborhood or have heard of cases;
iv.   The objectives of Session 2 discussed - To make a competent assessment of personal risk of infection;
v.   The purpose and methods of the self administered questionnaire explained;
vi.   Item by item discussion of some implications of various responses on the questionnaire;
vii.   Personal testimonies/reflections on the impact of the questionnaire – voluntary;
viii.   Is anyone truly "not at risk" of HIV infection given the wide range of links between sexual and other life style issues such as alcohol use, frequent separation from spouse or regular partners and opportunities for forming casual sexual relationships and the complications introduced by sexual networking;
ix.   What are the short and medium term implications of risk perceptions to the individual?

The sessions required considerable skills in managing group discussion in such a way that no one is exposed to ridicule. The pace of the discussion could often not be predicted, requiring occasional prompting by the session facilitator (In most cases the Principal Investigator) to keep discussions focussed. In some clinics, though, particular individuals had the disposition to draw others out by being open about their own self-risk assessment. At other sessions, a segment of the participants with similar background turn their risk assessment into a group within a group analysis with other participants feeding into the discussions with their own perceptions of the segment.

Whatever the dynamics of the first of these two sessions, towards the end, the participants usually clamoured for information on how to avoid the logical consequences of their sexual risk taking. This direction took the group towards the third stage of the 4-stage framework when information sharing was paramount.

Stage 3: If I am at risk? Give me the information and resources to reduce, modify or escape the logical outcome of risk taking.

It is at this stage of providing knowledge for risk reduction and behaviour modification that the conventional IEC approaches of the health belief models have excelled. A mixture of health talks, condom use demonstration, tips on managing condom use and other sexual negotiation and information on sources of services, clarification, voluntary counselling and testing, meets the needs of most participants. In addition, the participants are given hand outs and some have access to other reading materials and information. Clarification is then provided on apparent differences in their own sources and those provided within the fourth and fifth session of the series.

Although spouses were usually aware of the information provided at this stage from their family planning clinic contacts, nearly all the male partners were less well informed, if at all. Consequently, a prior decision was made that in order to assist males' learning and internalization of the information, the spouses would be invited to join them in the fifth and subsequent session. The hope was that by the end of the fourth session, the males would be comfortable enough about the group meetings and about the objectives and methods that they would not object to their spouses (client or non client of the DP clinics) sharing their experiences.

The suggestion to have the spouses join the sessions came at the end of the 3rd session from one of the Ibadan groups (PPFN Ibadan). Their justification was that their female partners/spouses were surprised and curious about the feedback the males gave them after the first two sessions. They wanted to know how the males suddenly became interested in family planning issues. The insinuation was that their spouses now felt that they too might be translating their newfound interest in family planning and AIDS prevention into promiscuity - a reversal of the "family planning corrupts" theme males used against FP.

The wide range of materials and resources involved at the third stage required that a multi-disciplinary team be put together to deliver the various components of the stage:

i.   Review of the self risk assessment session;
ii.   Implications of risks taken by relevant others - spouses, regular partners, teenage children and the wider community;
iii.   The purpose of the third stage with focus on information sharing;
iv.   Introduction to the concept of DP;
v.   DP as AIDS prevention strategy and related gender issue;
vi.   Introduction to the male and female condoms;
vii.   Demonstration of the condoms;
viii.   Scrutiny of female condom;
ix.   Using a pelvic model for a "Hands on" involvement with male insertion of female condom;
x.   Negotiating skills;
xi.   Drama sketches on issues of risk taking, condom negotiation and decision options;
xii.   Information on female condom distribution policy;
xiii.   IEC distribution.

In general this third stage required three 2-hour sessions. The arrival of spouses required that an overview of the first and second stages be given to the mixed group, so that the spouses could participate fully. The male partners were given the task of making summary presentations on what had been achieved by the group prior to the arrival of some of the spouses. The presentations of some husbands at these sessions revealed the changes in their knowledge and attitude in the course of the previous four meetings and came as a complete surprise to their spouses.

Stage 4: How do I have the motivation, resources and power to put all the knowledge into practice?

During the final stage of the 4-stage framework, the wealth of information and education material on how to prevent infection does not translate into actual change of patterns of behaviour unless the individual, couple or group has the motivation, resources and the negotiating power to put their knowledge into practice. This was the traditional explanation of the knowledge-behaviour gap pervading the translation of family planning knowledge into practice (Adeokun et al., 2004). Conventional IEC approaches to BCC also find the three previous stages easier and less confrontational. Consequently, this stage was usually the most difficult and protracted to realize.

In the Yoruba cultural setting, in which all of the current DP sub-projects are being implemented, the gender in-equity in sexual, reproductive health and family life between the sexes constitute the major barrier to the narrowing of the knowledge-behaviour gap. The central problem is the dominant role that males play in the life of females. The conventional concept of male involvement was to make males responsive to reproductive health issues essentially by providing them with the necessary information.

In contrast, the male group sessions focused on the male vulnerability to infections and addressed the altruism of sexual health as a secondary consideration. The new knowledge gained by males put them on the defensive as to the level of personal risks they face and the dangers they pose to relevant others. This is a form of role reversal between the sexes. The reluctant male debutante in the field of family planning and promotion of dual protection were turned, within a few months into advocates of safer sex and AIDS prevention. This was not out of consideration for the welfare of wives and children, but out of a patently selfish motive to stay alive, given what they then knew about the epidemic.

Language of communication

The major differential between the groups is the level of literacy and comfort with communications in the English language. Consequently all sessions were conducted in Yoruba. This is the mother tongue or second language for every member of the group.

Uniformity of facilitation

The sessions were 90% facilitated by the Principal Investigator. This served two purposes. It allowed uniformity in the presentation of materials and the management of discussions. Second, it allowed the necessary changes to be made to subsequent sessions on the basis of the immediate feedback from previous sessions. The use of video recording in some sessions was carefully planned with the group so that there was no occasion of grandstanding or exaggeration in the views expressed by either the males or their spouses. Some of the verbal information provided in some of the sessions has been validated with some of the findings from quantitative surveys on issues relating to AIDS prevention and sexual negotiation in the end of intervention general population survey.

RESULTS

Three separate issues are taken up in this section on results. The first relates to the performance of the males on the BCC programme. How much did they appreciate the reality of the AIDS epidemic? How competent was their risk awareness? And did they record any changes in attitude and behaviour? The indicators for some of this evaluation issues include the regularity of attendance at the session.

The second related to the findings from end of project KAP surveys that allowed some assessment of the impact of the intervention on the participants.

The third aspect of results rested on the qualitative assessment of the impact and outcomes of the intervention on the males as well as on some of the spouses who were present in the second phase of the intervention. Such assessments were obtained from wrap-up focus groups held at the end of intervention in which both males and their

spouses had an opportunity to reflect on the gains and problems of the male group programme. In a few of the discussions, the familiarity between all the participants and the project staff made the video taping of discussions easy and unrehearsed.
Performance of Males on BCC programme

Attendance at sessions

One major concern about the project design was that it hinged on the level of cooperation of males with the demands of the programme activities. It was doubted if attendance would be regular enough and in sufficient numbers to justify the efforts in human and material resources. This fear turned out to be largely unfounded. It must be stated that there were no major incentives to make people attend. For example, the transport allowance to defray the cost of attending the meeting was the local currency equivalent of $1.50 (one dollar, fifty cents). Because of the timing of the meetings in the afternoon and the 2-hour duration, a bottle of soft drink was provided to each participant at meetings. This choice of afternoons was theirs as it allowed participants to make an initial appearance at their respective places of work, attend to customers or reschedule appointments, before attending the sessions.

It was this factor of not staying away from work that created problems for some members. Those in the service trades such as tailors, barbers, and motor mechanics who depend on "walk-in" clientele found it difficult to turn away such clients or reschedule appointment. In effect, some delays in making up numbers were often recorded. But once the numbers were satisfactory, the members generally devoted the 2-hour needed to each session. The waiting time for some was taken up by informal discussions with project staff on aspects of previous sessions or in viewing video clips on various topics on HIV/AIDS and reproductive health.

There were very rare instances in which labour unrest or strikes by transport workers prevented a few individuals arriving on time or not attending. Those affected by such events were mostly civil servants, some of whom lived at some distance from the clinics close to their place of work.

Yet the pattern and regularity of attendance was one of the most impressive indicators of the level of commitment of the members to the programme. Once at the meeting, there was usually a palpable urgency to get as much done within the two hours as was possible. Discussions were lively and at times carried beyond the two-hour session. It was clear also that such discussions were carried over into their trade groups, since feedbacks were given that some of their friends and workplace colleagues, hearing what they were doing, would like to join in the sessions. Their promises that they would regularly "step down" their knowledge and that outreach activities will be conducted in their local groups, were the consolations to such colleagues.

RESPONSES TO THE 4 STAGES

Stage 1 (Session 1): Raised awareness of HIV/AIDS risk

At the beginning of the second session of the series, the participants gave some immediate feedbacks on reactions to the very first session. The feedbacks came from personal and reported experiences. In one of the male groups, a participant reported that since the first session he did not have the courage to continue his prevailing level of sexual activity and multiple sexual partnerships. The video clip showing the ravages of untreated or inadequately treated STIs and clips of individual Nigerians living with HIV/AIDS as well as the clear message of the link between having multiple sexual partners and risk of HIV infection was found convincing. Another participant reported the noticeable drop in the flirting habits of one of his colleagues at work. Perhaps a negative response was that of one member of a group who reportedly dropped out after the first session because he felt that, given the impact of just one session, the programme could end up dissuading him from further womanizing.

Stage 2 (Sessions 2 to 4): Making competent risk assessment

The result of the risk assessment in Session 2 was based on a socio-economic and life style questionnaire completed by the participants. Some of the items were innocuous enough and the discussions at the first sessions had not been detailed enough to raise anxieties about answering the questions. Most were also unaware of the implications of some of the answers they provided until the series of responses were reviewed. Since the anonymity of respondents was also maintained, everybody felt comfortable with the risk assessment exercise. They were all made aware that participation in the exercise was voluntary and that comments of personal experience depended on the readiness of the individual to share their experiences. As it turned out, all the participants present at the second session freely participated in the risk assessment. They also stated that it was unusual and interesting

Demographic variables and risk taking

According to the attendance register, 68 males participated in the risk assessment. The highlights of the findings can be summarized in the following terms:

In terms of the risks associated with the demographic variables of age and marital status, the following observations were made. The age ranged from 25 to 68. Given the decline in the frequency of sexual activity, as one grows older, the risk of STIs will show similar difference. Although participants were either married or in regular unions, they agreed that age is a predictor of the likelihood of the individual engaging in extramarital affairs.

Next attention was turned to the likely influence of type of marriage on sexual activity. It was pointed out that for the 5 single male participants who were not married, coping with their sexual desires was an issue. Of the 67 married males, 88% have one wife. However, the participants pointed out that those with many wives are not likely to be as promiscuous as those with one wife. The latter may be looking for variety in their sexual life. The banter with which the discussions were carried on indicated the level of acceptability of male infidelity in most of Yoruba society.

Economic and life style variables and risks

The combination of education level, occupation and opportunity to travel away from home was seen as a vital predictor of the risk taking among males and among females too, as some were eager to point out. In this connection, 69% of the participants stated that they had opportunities to make business trips away from home. Even when such opportunities do not exist, 71% of participants acknowledged that they regularly went out with male friends on social outings. Such outings were usually in the evening and some involved visits to public houses such as hotels and beer parlours. It was freely acknowledged in discussions that such outings could facilitate extramarital affairs.

Smoking and drinking were seen as dimensions of social acceptance. However, less than 5% of the participants smoked. Under a third (29%) drank any alcohol. Of the 21 males who drank alcohol, one in five did so regularly while the rest do so occasionally. It was pointed out in the risk assessment discussions that alcohol has the effect of loosening control, particularly at social events. The problem with alcohol consumption was with deciding when one had had enough. All agreed that alcohol consumption tended to make people amorous.

Sexual habits and risk of infection

After discussing these opening risk issues, attention was then turned to the number of multiple sexual partners reported in the survey. Participants were asked if they were sexually active in the month since the previous session. 91.7% were active. When asked the number of sexual partners they had in the interval, 8 individuals did not respond to the question. Of the 52 sexually active males who responded, 92% reported one partner. The remaining 9 individuals reported between 2 and 5 sexual partners. The discussion that followed reflected on what the group knew of the link between number of partners and risk of HIV infection. Consequently, the question on condom use was seen as addressing the concerns that might attach to having many partners.

Out of the 66 who were sexually active in the previous month, 26 (39%) used condoms; the rest did not. Nearly all those who used condoms used male condom. Only one male reported the use of a female condom. 57% used condom with their spouses, 31% with girl friends and one individual reported use of condom with a prostitute. The range of sexual behaviour reported in the risk assessment is outstanding for two reasons. The risk assessment came after the awareness creation session. Yet the link between sexual activity and risk of HIV infection did not put most respondents off going through the risk assessment exercise. In addition, the assurance given to participants that the discussion will not focus on individuals' answers but on implications of various characteristics reported appeared to have been accepted.

Attention was drawn to other sources of exposure to risk such as sharing of skin piercing objects such as razors. The link between such exposure and risk of blood-based infection was readily appreciated.

Response to new information and synergy with other AIDS prevention activities

To close the discussions on risk assessment, the participants were finally asked about their IEC exposure previous to the group sessions. Nearly all (91.7%) heard radio jingles about HIV/AIDS prevention before the group sessions began. Just under two-thirds (65.3%) had attended an AIDS prevention campaign somewhere in the city in the previous month. These responses point firmly to the symbiosis and synergies created between the male involvement intervention and other AIDS prevention initiatives within the city. This access of group members to other information sources ruled out the classic outcome evaluation of the impact of specific interventions. This does not detract from the central thesis of the sequence of processes leading from awareness to behaviour change in response to a health challenge.

Stage 3: Acquisition of knowledge and skills for risk reduction

Of the four stages the third is the conventional focus in IEC activities. Ignorance is often the basis of exposure to risk. Consequently, it is argued, once given the information, then all will be well with the subject. Development and distribution of IEC materials and other multimedia activities are carried out with the sole aim of saturating the target population with the necessary information.

In the male group intervention, the third stage was no different in methods from those employed in other stages. But the delivery of materials was not only multimedia it was multi-disciplinary. The team was made up of health educators and health providers who demonstrated the use of condom. Print and video materials were also used. Role play to illustrate some of the patterns of behaviour which should be encouraged or discouraged, as the case may be, was also employed.

It was on the central position of knowledge in the process of behaviour change and the need to have both male and female sexual partners participate in the acquisition of that knowledge that led to the invitation to spouses to join the fifth and subsequent sessions of the male group intervention. Having some of the couples present allowed some of the dynamics of condom use, for example, to be discussed by both sexes in an interactive way.

Stage 4 (Sessions 7 & 8): Translating knowledge into practice through negotiation and gender equity in sexual and reproductive health

The gains of Stage 3 in terms of knowledge and skill acquisition by participants of both sexes laid the ground for the implementation of some of the programmes making up the fourth and final stage. There were four elements of empowerment identified in the application of sexual and reproductive health knowledge into action. First, was discussion of the benefits and costs of any sexual activity in which people engage. Condom use, multiple sexual partnership alcohol abuse were all activities people carry out because they get some pleasure from them. By encouraging a free flowing group discussion on some of these activities the participants were able to identify for themselves some of the hidden costs to the individuals and significant others. Examples include the realization that most pleasures are not essential for survival, that there was some money and other emotional resources to be devoted to the pleasure, and that some pleasures exert their cost in physical and health consequences.

The second element of the final stage was devoted to the extent to which exogenous factors constraint the individual in putting knowledge to use. Participants were chosen to prepare and make presentations at a subsequent session on such topics as the cultural factors affecting or condoning patterns of sexual behaviour among the sexes. Authors of such presentations were encouraged to be as subjective or objective as they wish. A dialogue followed such presentations drawing out the extent to which such factors may be static or dynamic.

A third element of empowerment was the strength of character a person brought to the behaviour change enterprise. It was openly acknowledged in discussions that the ability to resist temptation of the sexual kind varied significantly. Some suggestion was made about having multiple sexual patterns being habit forming. But in as much as some smokers can give up smoking and others cannot, the importance of character must be recognized. As to what formed character, there were a variety of suggestions. Family background, parental influence and religious beliefs were some of the components of character formation discussed.

The final element in the empowerment sessions consisted of the review of relationships between males and females, husbands and wives, the old and the young, the powerful and the weak, and such other relationships that lend themselves to the exploitation of subordinates by their superiors. The discussion focused on three sexual behaviour patterns that have their origins in these power relations. Sexual harassment in schools and colleges, males' extra-marital affairs against the wishes of their spouses and the use of commercial sex workers were discussed as dimensions of male-female power relations.

In the end, it was agreed that of all the elements of empowerment, the character issue was the most significant in being able to put knowledge to practice. The understanding between couples, their ability to discuss issues of interest could contribute to improvement in relationships. However, it was recognized that some of the gender issues were culturally rooted and only being slowly eroded by education.

IMPACT OF DUAL PROTECTION PROMOTION

Knowledge

The delivery of knowledge of HIV/AIDS prevention is one of the strong points of IEC activities. In this intervention, it was possible to record substantial increase in knowledge of channels of transmission and prevention among the male participants. This was consistent to the level of exposure two-thirds had prior to the intervention. However, far more relevant to AIDS control and management is what the reaction of the participants to those will be.

Knowledge of DP was higher among the females than among the males at 70.6% and 64.6% respectively. Those familiar with the concept were able to define what it connotes adequately. The method of recruitment of males, which resulted in some who had no spouses in the clinic and the similar inclusion of females who were spouse to such males, meant that some missed the crucial session 3 and 4 at which the basic concepts were discussed.

Attitude: stigma and tolerance of PLWHAs

The issues of stigma attached to HIV/AIDS and the extent to which participants will be tolerant was investigated. In the seven-item Stigma measures, the males were compared with their female spouses to see how each performed. The proportions claiming each statement to be true are shown on Table 6.1.

t appeared that there was greater convergence between males and their spouses with regards to tolerance of PLWHAs than on the stigma they attach to persons who were HIV infected. In general, the males showed a tendency towards a lower degree of stigmatization of PLWHAs than the spouses. It must be remembered that the males were the ones exposed to the longer period of BCC than the females.

HOW DIFFICULT IS BEHAVIOUR CHANGE?

Taking HIV Test as a major decision
It was possible to assess the degree of sexual behaviour change traceable to the intervention in the case of the decision to take an HIV test. The respondents were asked some direct questions about those changes in sexual and other behaviour patterns they made as a result of the male group initiative. Going for an HIV test represents a major decision.

Table 6.1: Reactions of male and females to stigma and tolerance of PLWH statement

STIGMA STATEMENTS:	Males	Fem.	Total
1. HIV infected persons are sexually loose	43.1	47.1	43.9
2. HIV infected persons are not useful to anyone	40.0	52.9	42.7
3. HIV infected persons are responsible for their problems	53.8	41.2	51.2
4. Mothers stand by their children whatever the condition	75.4	82.4	76.8
5. Public health providers are friendly with HIV infected	73.8	94.1	78.0
6. HIV infected persons should not be allowed to mix	40.0	64.7	45.1
7. HIV/AIDS is a punishment from God	21.5	17.6	20.7
TOLERANCE STATEMENTS			
1. Will sleep with HIV infected persons in the same room	52.3	52.9	52.4
2. Will visit those with HIV/AIDS in hospital	72.3	82.4	74.4
3. Will help carry someone dying of AIDS into ambulance	64.6	64.7	64.6
4. Will tell others if relative dies of AIDS after long illness	76.9	76.5	76.8
5. Some tribes are more tolerant of sick people than others	60.0	64.7	61.0
6. The better educated are more tolerant of PLWHA	50.8	64.7	53.7
7. Some religious people better able to look after PLWHA	49.2	64.7	52.4

Source: Project End of intervention questionnaire survey

It follows from a sense of doubt and a search for assurance. 13.8% of the 65 males claimed to have taken the HIV test as a direct result of the intervention. None of the 17 spouses interviewed reported taking the test. This pattern reflected the general impression of both sexes that males were more promiscuous than females. In addition, the males were the ones subjected to the more sustained programme of risk assessment and education for behaviour change. Some of the females were subjected to a personalized risk assessment within the counselling framework of FP clinics. A few had no previous contact with the FP clinics. Other measures of impact of the male group intervention showed less dramatic difference between the sexes or between the time of the risk assessment and the end of intervention survey.

Level of sexual activity

One area of interest in behaviour change is the sexual response to the increased awareness of the risk of unsafe sex. But the change in safe sex may be at the expense of unaltered level of sexual activity. At baseline out of 72 males, 66 were sexually active in the previous month, [26 (39%) of these used condoms; the rest did not]. At the end of intervention, the proportion reporting use of condom increase significantly to 61%.

Increased condom use

The focus on male cooperation with spouses in the adoption of dual protection took into account that the male condom remains the predominant barrier method of choice. The female condom was promoted as a viable supplement. In effect, the increases reported for both male and female condom use is a sign of behaviour change in the target population. There was no significant difference registered in the level of sexual activity reported by males at their risk assessment exercise and at end of intervention. However, male condom use increased from 39.3% among those sexually active at baseline to 61% at the end of intervention. Female condom use rose substantially from 4% of condom users at the risk assessment exercise in February 2002 to 13.8% and end of intervention six months later.

Number of sexual partners and use of condom

At the risk assessment exercise, 82.6% of sexually active males reported only one partner. The proportion at end of intervention was not significantly higher at 84.7%. The real progress was that the proportion of sexually active males who used condoms rose from 39.3% to 61%.

Table 6.2: Changes in social activities by end of intervention

Changes in social activities	At risk assessment	End of intervention	
	Males	Males	Spouses
Social club membership	41.7	69.2	58.8
Social outings	70.8	56.9	41.2
Business travel	69.4	58.5	23.5
Drink alcohol occasionally	(29.2)	(26.2)	0.0
Drink regularly	23.6	18.5	0.0

Source: Evaluation Survey Analysis.

Adjustments to social life

Both males and the spouses attending had an opportunity to report those specific changes they made to their social life in response to any of the components of the intervention. Information were obtained on the level of social drinking, going out with friends or membership of a social club, and opportunities for going on business travel in the risk assessment exercise. At the end of the intervention, these same profiles were revisited.

From the responses it will be observed that there were some changes and that some behaviour patterns remained immutable. For example, club membership, which is a way of traditional life, and a form of social organisation are seen to show some increase. It was on this premise that the Yoruba like working in groups, that the idea of setting up the male group was based.

Some other items of risk exposure were added at end of intervention survey. They included previous exposure to blood transfusion. 10.8% received blood in the past. Most did so over a year before the date of interview. Exposure to therapeutic injections was widespread with more than 80% of both males and females reporting previous injections. One third of these individuals had an injection within the year 2002. All these non-sexual activities give an indication of the residual risks of HIV infection that do not feature directly in most sex-oriented AIDS prevention education.

OTHER SELF REPORTED BEHAVIOUR CHANGES

Abstinence

The choice of abstinence is limited within marriage. Since most of the males were either married or in regular unions, it came as a surprise that abstinence was mentioned by 11 of the 65 male participants and by one of the 16 female participants. One cultural situation that prompts abstinence in marriage is when the woman attains the status of grandmother whilst still within her reproductive ages. This is not uncommon given the extent of early marriages still occurring in Nigeria as well as in Yoruba society.

Avoiding casual sex

The prevalence of extra-marital affairs among males is an issue that the prevention and control of AIDS epidemic must contend with (Messersmith et. al., 2000). Documenting the phenomena in terms of number of sexual partners was made difficult by the existence of substantial levels of polygamy. However, by their own report, 37 of 65 males and 5 of 17 females cited avoiding casual sex as a response they made to the intervention.

HIV PREVENTION SELF EFFICACY

Against the background of the detailed programme of 4-stage framework of behaviour modification attempted with the groups, the degree of HIV prevention self-efficacy achieved is a sign of the feasibility of the approach. At the time of planning male involvement, the awkwardness of male presence at the clinics was mentioned. The low level of inter-spousal communication on sexual activity or fertility decisions was also recognized and a barrier to male involvement in family planning, sexual and reproductive health. However, after months of making appearances at the clinics,

Table 6.3: HIV Prevention Self-efficacy

99% can discuss AIDS with sexual partner

94% can ask FP providers for condoms if they needed them

89% can ask if a sexual partner has an STD

82% can ask if sexual partner had another sexual partner in the past 12 months

68% can refuse to have sex if the partner does not agree to condom use

there was a noticeable improvement in the general inter-personal communication skills of some of the participants. Apparently, these skills were extended into their other interactions. Table 6.3 shows the indicators of HIV prevention self-efficacy among the males. These indicators speak for themselves. The point worth making is that restraint in sexual matters is not a norm among Yoruba males.

DISCUSSION

What went well?

a)   Working as a group in adoption of innovation

The evidence in the literature is strong that group dynamics works well with introduction of innovations including those encouraging behaviour change (Kebaabetswe and Noor, 2002). On this occasion, the group format served the purpose of a mutual support group for males who were going into the unknown territory of participation in reproductive health programming.

b)   Making a habit of learning

Another well established learning principle is that if people make a habit of learning through regular contacts with information and education platform, they take the content more seriously than in sporadic learning opportunity. By making the group sessions regular, attendance was strengthened and monitoring learning and reinforcing it was made simpler.

The content and methods of the learning process were also planned with a view of making it appeal to a wide range of educational as well as socioeconomic background. The local language formed the means of communication. This also forced people to think deeply about concepts some of which are strange to the language.

c)   Self-interest is a good starting point for male involvement

One of the major observations on the project is the extent to which the males were propelled by self-interest into participation. Some observed that given the potential for male promiscuity and the reality of the HIV/AIDS epidemic, the one survival strategy was for males to change their sexual behaviour or at least take the recommended precaution of using condoms.

The addition of a spousal participation in the last stages of the series helped some males to take their new and strange enthusiasm for safer sex to their surprised and amazed spouses.   A spectacular instance was caught on video. A spouse reported that the husband was coming home early from work, returning with more income and being more attentive to the needs of the family. The altruism for the welfare of the family is an extension of the understanding of the individual male that the welfare of the family is an extension of their own welfare.

d)   Once emboldened males can motivate males

It emerged from the early stages that once the males were given the information and education to protect that self interest, they were willing to share the information with colleagues who did not have the opportunity to participate in the group sessions. The more outgoing characters among the male members turned out to be the more adventurous in getting the message to others.

Some limitations

a)   Behaviour change communication is expensive

The series is demanding of human resource inputs in the formation of the first group of peer promoters. The development of the IEC materials, the assurance of standards in the delivery of messages and the facilitation of groups require a sustained attention to planning the details of each session so that it builds on previous ones. The health education content is sophisticated and requires documentation and further analysis to appreciate the impact of this 4-stage framework intervention.

b)   Demand is high for technical support

The intervention has been equally demanding of technical support for its continuation. The multimedia IEC materials require some equipment and support staff for effective use. In effect, the male promoters may, in turn, be able to start their own groups, but they will require some technical assistance if such secondary groups are to be sustained.

CONCLUSION

Lessons learnt

Adopting the 4-stage framework as the health belief model to the design of IEC intervention for behaviour change was something of a gamble to begin with. Will males take time off from bread winning to attend all sessions? Will they wish to discuss their personal life in front of others? Will they find behaviour change communication intrusive and resist? Those were the nagging questions. On the flip side, the advantage of group forum for encouraging adoption of innovation has been documented (Kebaabetswe, P. and Noor, Kathleen F., 2002). In as much as this sustained approach has not been tried before in the Ibadan clinical setting, the novelty was a plus. The very targeting of males was also a novelty. But the greatest strength was assembling the range of IEC materials (video material, print and drama) with which to sustain the 8-session programme. In the meantime the groundswell of interest in the electronic media meant that the target population was receiving reinforcement of its learning from other sources.

The evidence that the gamble carried limited risk could be seen in the commitment and sustained attendance and participation of the group members at all clinics. Although there were some demographic and social differences between members of each group, those differences turned to an advantage in the range and richness of discussions at the sessions. For example there were more than 20 different occupations represented among the 65 males while the females were more clustered on four major occupations (trading, tailoring, teaching and civil service).

The high level of commitment was obtained primarily by the importance of the topic of discussion and the interest of everyone in self-improvement and preservation. In spite of the difficult economic situation and pressure on Nigerians, incentives did not play a major part in that commitment. The token transport allowance was more an effort to supplement a suitable travel mode than to compensate for any loss of trade which some of the participants surely suffered in the course of the intervention.

It is possible that the absence of language barrier in tackling sexual, moral and ethical issues with the predominantly Yoruba group was an advantage. It is equally conceivable that the PI being a Yoruba elder, made communication easier than would have been the case if the facilitator had been younger than the participants. The same could be said that the PI, being a male, was an advantage. The behaviour communication series demanded an understanding of the male point of departure so that changes advocated were seen as logical rather than a critique of a way of life of males or of Yoruba culture. After the recognition of logic, the recognition of the harmful impact of norms, values and culture is easy to handle.

Two unresolved issues were raised by the series. The first is how to sustain the male interest in reproductive health issues in the absence of any radical modification or expansion in male relevant services made available in the family planning clinics. The other is how to make the males peer educators in their own rights.

In answer to the first, the male groups have been quick in recognizing the educational aspect of the series and the benefits to themselves and others. The new knowledge expands their ability to access other sexual and reproductive health services in both the public and private sector in spite of the lack of similar services in the FP setting. The other beneficiaries of the series are the providers, who in spite of being members of the opposite sex gained in acceptability because they were seen as source of information and further clarification of RH problems males bring to their attention. The providers also learnt in practical terms that the presence of the male partners could be accommodated within the limitations of existing structures and services. The other female clients not involved in the male group intervention were fascinated that some spouses were comfortable and empowered enough to involve their husbands in the behaviour change venture in their sexual life.

The issue of male group members transforming later into peer educators was resolved very early in the series. Without any prompting from project staff, all the groups appointed their own leaders at the very first session. This may be a Yoruba culture thing. But it does help in giving the group a sense of continuity. For example, the secretary kept minutes of sessions and absentees send in apologies. In other groups, the chosen leaders served as contacts to the others when the occasion demanded.

Another aspect of the formal status of the participants is the promise that all those who attended a minimum of six sessions, with attendance in each of the four stages of self preservation as the adopted model came to be known will be given a Peer Educator certificate of ARFH affirming that the individual had gone through the equivalent of a PE course.

Without doubt, it is the empowerment of the knowledge gained that propelled the peer education zeal of the participants. After the first session, the temptation was high to bring in new members. But given the experimental nature of this attempt, such new members were discouraged. Instead the situation developed where the group members were able to step down the knowledge and information gained to smaller groups in their neighbourhood, work places and in social or faith based settings.

CHAPTER 7
PROMOTING HIV PREVENTION IN AT RISK POPULATIONS

INTRODUCTION

At the end of the promotion of the DP in the six FP clinics, the feasibility of three of the four stages of behaviour change necessary for the adoption of DP by women was well established. But with the imperfections surrounding the last stage of behaviour change, additional effort was required to overcome the difficulties women faced in adopting barrier methods in general and the FC in particular. The situation was further complicated by the association which was now well established that the renewed interest in barrier methods was in the context of the HIV/AIDS epidemic.

The involvement of male partners of the FP clients in the DP promotion resulted in the validation of the assumption that if men constituted the constraint to barrier methods, they were necessary for its removal. By turning the focus of the justification of DP from the welfare of women to the self preservation of the males the focus of attention of males turned from the pleasure motive of sexual activity and promiscuity to the urgency of assuring self survival by acknowledging the seriousness of the threats they faced if they continued with their ongoing patterns of sexual behaviour and risk taking. The Male Involvement Group (MIG) programme removed all doubts about the rigorous logic and replicable nature of the 4-stage framework. In effect, it was time to attempt a general population introduction of the BBC model so as to reach more people. The quality of the programme outcomes also demonstrated the importance of employing the model as a robust tool of HIV prevention. For this to be achieved, the main vulnerable groups and drivers of the epidemic had to be reached with this effective tool of BCC.

The Most at Risk Populations (MARPS) are a variety of population groups who through their activities expose themselves and others to the risk of STIs including HIV. The groups vary in size and in their potential impact on the spread of the HIV epidemic. The more frequently cited populations are Commercial Sex workers (CSW), Intravenous drug users (IDUs) and Men having Sex with Men (MSM). However, the incidence and accessibility of these risky behaviours vary from country to country. In addition, focus on these groups draws attention away from the more public health related activities of others who are more in number and have the potential to contribute significantly to the spread of their HIV epidemic. These other groups can be described as At Risk Population (ARPS).

The At Risk Populations (ARPS) included in the APIN/ARFH projects were those whose behaviour actively aided the spread of the epidemic if they were not provided with the preventive education and behaviour modification prior to their full scale entry into the sexually active population group. In the group were out of school youths whose daily activities included the high potential for involvement in transactional sexual activity as well as some form of payment for sexual interactions. Others were in-school youths who were on the threshold of sexual debut or indulgence in sexual activity and allied risk taking. The adult population in trading activities in market places also fall in the ARPS. The age composition of the population in the markets suggested that they were mostly in the sexually active age groups. Their socio-economic profile also suggested that they may not have adequate access to information on the epidemic. The other group among the ARPS were the clients of public or private health institutions some of whom were already showing up with sexually transmitted infections including HIV.

Contrary to the direct information, education and communication approach adopted for communication of the 4-stage framework to FP clients or to their male partners, a change in strategy was required for the scaling up of the outreach of the model to be achieved. Consequently, the targets of the projects were the intermediaries who were to be trained as 4-stage framework communicators so that they, in turn, can take segments of MARPS through the behaviour change processes. The outcome was the development of four sub-projects that addressed different approaches to AIDS prevention within Ibadan City and targeted different constituencies of the MARPS. The four APIN supported sub-projects respectively were titled:

1. Sexual Health Counsellors (In and out of school)
2. Market Agent Programme with focus on Male Involvement in Dual Protection
3. Integration of Dual Protection in General Practice

As the respective titles suggest, the first sub-projects worked through selected and trained sexual health counsellors located in secondary schools and among out of school youths. The market based sub-project worked through Market Agents selected from the markets, trained and deployed to promote DP and to focus on the proven involvement of male traders and clients in this approach to HIV prevention. And the third sub-project stayed within the health institution framework of earlier DP promotion projects but scaled up the promotion to 83 private clinics through selected and trained DP service providers from among the staff of the clinics.

The timing of the MARPS sub-projects (April 2001 to November 2002) was ideal for Oyo State for a number of reasons:
1. Although the first cases of HIV/AIDS were identified in the state, as well as in Nigeria, in 1986, whilst the national HIV prevalence had reached 5.4% by year 2000, Oyo State reached the relatively lower rate of 3.8%.
2. At less than 5% prevalence rate, the case could be made that initiating a number of AIDS prevention programmes that addressed behaviour change among major risk groups in the population was worth the effort, so that the

rate could remain low.

3. The enabling environment for AIDS prevention activities in the State was in part due to the presence of NGOs that were involved in on-going and complementary AIDS prevention programmes such as the promotion of Dual Protection in family planning clinics within Ibadan Metropolis and the implementation of the Extended Life Planning Education (ELPE) in public secondary schools.

The overall goal of the sub-projects was to provide information, education and communication to the major groups of population at risk of HIV infection in such a way as to encourage some behaviour change, as individuals and groups become familiar with the relative risks of the sexual norms they hold and the decisions they make. The aims and objectives of the respective sub-projects are as listed below.

1. Sexual Health Counsellors (In and out of school)

The two objectives for the youth sub-project were:

a) To increase their sexual health/HIV/AIDS awareness through a system of sexual health counselling provided by specially trained schools-based and community based trained counsellors; and

b) To train at least 2 counsellors per school and 2 community-based counsellors to educate, counsel and provide referral for sexual health problems to Youth Friendly Clinics in project schools or in PHC facilities.

2. Market Agent Programme with focus on Male Involvement in Dual Protection

The two objectives were:

a) To encourage HIV prevention awareness and behaviour change in general population groups who come in regular contact with market agents; and

b) To have market agents trained in HIV education and counselling skills and the distribution of barrier methods.

3. Integration of Dual Protection in Private General Medical Practice

The overall aim of the sub-project was to sensitize the private health sector to the control and management of HIV/AIDS. This was achieved through the following objectives:

a) Re-awaken the consciousness of the private medical and health services community to HIV/AIDS reality and prevention.

b) Increase knowledge and strengthen counselling skills of private health providers in HIV/AIDS prevention in the participating facilities.

c) Integrate social marketing of condom (Male/Female) into service provision.

In the rest of the chapter the materials and methods of the three sub-projects will be discussed in the context of attaining the staged behaviour changes. Results of the evaluation of the sub-projects are also presented. They revealed the substantive changes that were made by the intermediaries [peer educators, market agents and private sector health providers] as well as by the ultimate beneficiaries during the interventions.

SUMMARY OF THE THREE SUB-PROJECTS

In this section brief details of the actual programmes and activities in each of the three groups are provided to show how they relate to the overall purpose of attaining behaviour change from whatever the standpoint of individuals and groups on the HIV/AIDS epidemic. These details form the background to the evaluation section which immediately follows.

TARGETING IN- AND OUT-OF-SCHOOL YOUTH AND THEIR COMMUNITIES

The training of school teachers, students and community-based peer educators in sexual health and HIV/AIDS counselling and behaviour change motivation was proposed as a way of addressing the needs of in- and out-of-school youths in the participating institution, communities and facilities. The training was based on the manuals that were developed on earlier DP projects as well as those which were used in the implementation of the Extended Life Planning Education project supported by DfID in Oyo State public secondary schools which began in 1998. The 10-day training consisted of the following elements discussed in the ensuing paragraphs.

Both students and teachers were trained in peer education and counselling skills and provided with IEC materials and a simple documentation system to keep records of their activities. The programme was supervised and monitored through a combination of monthly meetings of educators and counsellors and occasional school visits by supervising project staff.

Because of the differences in educational background, separate training sessions were conducted for the out-of-school peer educators using the same manuals and materials but using the local language as the medium of communication where necessary.

Because of this prior exposure of Oyo State public secondary schools' population to the project of Extended Life Planning Education (ELPE), the activities of the peer educators and teacher sexual health counsellors had a cumulative effect in promoting AIDS prevention, awareness and allied behaviour change among the students. Baseline information for that programme (ELPE Chart Book 1999) had established that high levels of sexual activity, early age of sexual debut and poor knowledge coupled with low use of condoms among secondary school population, created a dangerous setting for the potential explosion of sexually transmitted infections (STIs) including HIV/AIDS. Consequently, the sub-project counsellors assisted youths with their personal risk assessment, risk reduction and prevention as well as provided them referral for reproductive health problems including STIs and HIV/AIDS.

The in-school programme was linked to the out-of-school component through the organisation of joint outreach activities between the in-school and out-of-school peer educators. At the end of nearly a year of operations, a general population survey was carried out in all parts of the metropolis so that the project LGAs could be compared with the non-project LGAs. In addition, sample survey interviews were carried out in schools among peer educators and among non-peer educators as a means of tracking the patterns of knowledge and attitude and behaviour changes that could be related to the project intervention.

Attainment of goals of Sexual Health Educator programme

a) Criteria for selection of school, student and teacher peers – re ELPE

The decision was taken that with 85 public secondary schools in Ibadan City, the selection of some and exclusion of others was likely to be problematic. Most of the state schools that benefitted from the Expanded Life Planning Education project in Ibadan metropolis, for which ARFH provided technical assistance to the State government, were again included in the APIN sub-project. This decision produced the total number of 83 schools involved in the sub-project. But contrary to the phased implementation of that ELPE project over a number of years, the short span of the APIN supported project and the focus of the intervention precluded such phasing. In effect all programmes and activities for the schools were carried out at the same time.

On the basis of the information obtained from the baseline survey for the ELPE, the selection of students and teachers for peer education and RH counselling training was based on the criteria that served the purpose of the ELPE. The process had inputs from students, staff, and principal in the respective schools. The tendency was for students in leadership position to be included and some volunteering on the basis of the letter of invitation to training sent to the schools through the principals.

b) Training and the production of calendar from IEC sessions

149 students made up of nearly equal numbers of both sexes drawn from 43 public secondary schools were involved in 10-day training workshop. The training gave the participants the ability to discuss the process of HIV infection, course and prevention; plan and conduct IEC activities; refer clients to relevant level of care and keep accurate but simple record of peer educational activities. In addition the participants were expected to take on the lessons of the 4-stage framework for their own personal

protection. A similar training workshop was organized for the 60 youth and 60 adult community based peer educators to supplement the work of the in-school PE's.

During the training of the in-school group, the IEC planning session include the conceptualization and realization of their own messages. The students worked in groups and came out with some 30 different posters. A peer review process of the posters produced the identification of the 12 most apt messages. These were incorporated into Year 2002 project calendar.

c) MIS and referral card and diary

One of the innovations on the APIN/ARFH sub-project, based on lessons learnt on earlier projects was the simplification of records of daily activity upon which the evaluation of performance of each PE was based. The record included only the essential elements of what activities each PE carried out. These were "one on one" counselling, health talks on AIDS prevention given to groups, distribution of IEC materials, referral of contacts for further information or services, and records of problems encountered by PE.

d) Monthly meetings to review peer education and teacher counselling and referral activities

Coordinating the activities of nearly 170 PE's and about the same number of teachers required that avenues be created for regular sharing of experiences among and between the two sets of in-school educators. Separate monthly meetings were arranged from August 2001 to June 2002 at which both groups of students and teachers were able to focus on the issues relating to the implementation of the peer education and counselling activities in their schools. The meetings were structured in such a way as to bring to light the factors which facilitated the smooth operations as well as the challenges they faced in their respective schools. The meetings also allowed the exchange of ideas as to how such problems can be resolved.

At these meetings short question and answer sessions were devoted to what behaviour changes the peers and the staff counsellors have observed in the school population that could be attributed to the intervention. The participants also discussed the phases of behaviour modification that they noticed among the school population

Achievements among in- and out-of-school youth

Although the in-school peer educators functioned primarily in schools, they were active in their local communities as well. The explanation of this dichotomy is simple. All the secondary schools were day-schools. Consequently, peer educators spent around half their waking hours in school and half among their out-of-school counterparts in other activities which included, learning a trade or taking part in income generating activities. It was in this context that they were able to attain high volumes of peer education. Over the course of the 10 months of project intervention, the in-school PE's were able to counsel an average of 100 individuals per month. This produced a monthly average total of 14,000 contacts. Cumulatively, the 10-month period produced over 140,000 contacts. Although there may be some repeat contacts as PE's follow up with some students, the amount of coverage attained by them was consistent with the large secondary school population, the opportunities to supplement in school activities with out-of-school activities and the enthusiasm with which the PE's operated on the sub-project.

The combined population of the 85 secondary schools was over 250,000. Even if all the activities of the PE's were in school, it means that over half the school population was reached. In actual fact, since they were also active out-of-school, the proportion of the school population reached was probably lower.

The distribution of IEC materials attained by the PE's was close to a ratio of two handouts per contact. This was consistent with the variety of IEC materials produced in both English and Yoruba and the preference of some contacts to have one of each or to choose a variety of messages available.

With regards to the issue of referring contacts to other sources of information or services, the in-school PE's sent about 1 percent of their contacts to health facilities after providing initial HIV prevention education. The reasons for such referrals were often related to STIs, additional information on AIDS prevention and occasionally, people asking to be put in touch with testing facilities for HIV. This aspect of the work of peer educators demonstrated that the move from the stage of awareness creation was followed up with effective assistance in assessing vulnerability among those counselled.

During the post intervention evaluation, of the 653 respondents in the school survey, 17.6 percent cited student PEs and 17.6% cited teachers as their source of information on HIV/AIDS. Together, these account for nearly a third of the respondents. The proportion citing handbills and posters stood at one in five. One in eight cited friends as their source of information. Because of the possibility for multiple answers, the combined effect of the peer education and RH counselling may well be higher than the sum of those who cited PE's and counsellors. Some of those who cited "friends" as source of information may have included their PE friends in this category. The main issue was that the effectiveness of the educators and counsellors in triggering behaviour change in the target population was clearly demonstrated.

When other measures of PEs impact were considered, the extent of their contribution was more precisely estimated. For example, out of the 653 teachers and students interviewed in the school based survey, a third (36.4%) claimed to have participated in enlightenment campaigns organized on HIV/AIDS in the past year. There were those who cited both PEs and Counsellors as sources of information but did not attend enlightenment campaigns. There was also some overlap between those who received information from both PEs and Counsellors. Another interesting assessment of the work of the two groups was their contribution to the decision to take an HIV test. Of the roughly one in ten (9.3%) of the respondents who had tested for HIV, about a third had contacts with both student educators and teacher counsellors.

It was obvious that the personal approach to behaviour change involved in peer education and RH counselling provided only a relatively short period of time during which to move those they target from awareness to risk assessment and from receiving information on HIV prevention to the initiation of important behaviour change decisions. In spite of this, deciding to go for the HIV test was a sign of major commitment to behaviour change. The proportion of students and teachers going for the HIV test was roughly equal while the proportion of males going for the test was significantly higher than the proportion of females. This was consistent with the understanding that the male were becoming aware that their sexual behaviour was making them prone to the risk of infection. This analysis was particularly applicable to the students among whom males were 1.5 times more likely to go for the test than female students. The ratio among male and female teachers who went for the HIV test was one to one.

Apart from the effects of the peer education and RH counselling on the student population, the most enduring features of their participation in the intervention was in terms of some of the values that these change agents took away from the exercise. These benefits included personal empowerment, improved self-efficacy and an awareness of the multiplier effect they can have on their colleagues.

Coping with peculiarities

The school based programme had limitations imposed by the assumption of resistance to the promotion of barrier methods on school premises. But this was more than made up by the enthusiasm that secondary schools, including those not in the project area were showing for AIDS prevention activities in terms of health talks, film shows and drama sketches. This sub-project staff participated, on request, in a number of such supplementary project activities.

The school calendar was disrupted significantly during the implementation of the sub-project. The flow over of students' and teachers' activities into the community was another compensation for the time lost in school-based interventions.

Discussion

One vital instrument of coordinating school based activities has been to work through the administrative framework. Logistics of distributing circulars for meetings, or informing principals and teachers of meeting was considerably facilitated by the advocacy to the Local Inspectors of Education (LIEs).

Employing groups sessions at which students and teachers from different schools can discuss issues improved the standards of performance among each cadre. Tips on problem solving were readily exchanged.

Conclusion to the in- and out-of-school youth sub-project

In conclusion, the school based intervention and the integration of a community element has been a major platform of reaching a very crucial age group in HIV/AIDS prevention activities. As some of them move on from the secondary schools, they will be taking with them some knowledge and skills which will come into use in the next crucial stage of their life spent in young adulthood and in another risk prone environment of the tertiary institutions.

Lessons learnt on the in- and out-of-school youth sub-project

When students and out-of-school youth work in groups, there was spontaneity in their actions that revealed a level of innocence still retained in spite of the barrage of moral sapping information in the print and electronic media. Those who made it to being peer educators may certainly not be average students. They came to the training with a level of confidence and assurance that was augmented by the acquisition of new skills.

Policy impact

The advantages of the peer education approach were cumulative. Training a cadre of them added to existing pools generated on other activities. The more the schools involved, the greater the attention which the approach received in education and policy cycles.

PEER PROMOTION AGENTS IN FIVE IBADAN MARKETS

Introduction

The classification of the market based population of traders and clients as at risk of HIV infection was firmly based on the epidemiological information on the dynamics of the HIV/AIDS epidemic. Prior to the epidemic there were features of market places that encouraged or facilitated transactional sexual activities. Traditional markets based on sales of agricultural products involves the competition of mostly female traders for access to the farm products which were being provided mostly by male farmers who produced, albeit, with the entire family labour the farm products. In such a set up, the use of sex as exchange commodity encouraged some level of involvement with multiple sexual partners.

Given the limited familiarity with HIV basics among the market population at the early stages of the epidemic and the relatively low levels of prophylactic use of barrier methods among the market population, it was no surprise that they were recognized as most at risk of HIV infection early in the epidemic. Without the sales of farm products the women stood no chance of benefiting from the labour they contributed to farming and without conceding to the demands of the sexually adventurous males, their access to the products would be limited. To this conundrum must be added the prime position of males in traditional sexual mores. The fundamental problem, therefore, was to restructure the uneven power relations between males and females in the market setting so that behaviour can be more voluntary than coerced and so that the chances of behaviour modification for HIV prevention can have a better chance of success.

With the expansion of markets into sale of manufactured goods, the stranglehold of farmers on trading codes was diluted but not broken. In addition, this change produced a wider range of socio-economic profile in the population patronizing the market and introduced new power brokers into the access of traders to the manufactured goods which were predominantly controlled by male distributors at the factory level and by female retailers. Consequently the markets constitute an ideal setting in which the sexual negotiating strategies were put side by side with the economic bargaining strategies for which the Yoruba were noted. The dual protection concept was introduced into the context of sexual negotiation so that both sexes saw the advantage to themselves in encouraging the use of barrier methods. And the framework for behaviour modification again relied on the tried and tested 4-stage framework which had served the purpose of the promotion of DP and the involvement of male partners in the FP settings.

Under the APIN/ARFH sub-projects, a programme of HIV/AIDS prevention within 5 Ibadan market communities was implemented using a network of ten male and female stall owners as agents of change in each project market. After being recruited and trained, they created awareness, attitudes and behaviour modification and change necessary for HIV/AIDS prevention. This same strategy was tested with some success in the community-based delivery of Reproductive Health services in the 1980's. However, the focus shifted from the population control and family planning to involving males in the process of change in sexual negotiation which was considered as fundamental to restructuring the unequal powers between the sexes. Such male involvement was also a reflection of the rising sex ratio in the major markets with increasing male participation in the sale of manufactured products in the traditional market settings. In the past, the emphasis on sale of food items made markets a female dominated arena.

Selection of markets

For the market agent sub-project, six markets were selected within Ibadan metropolis.

The factors that influenced the selection included earlier participation of a market in some of the CBD programmes of ARFH in the late 1980s, approval of the market leadership to be involved in the project and to ensure the cooperation of the various sub-groups of trade associations within the market. At the end of the selection process two markets from the CBD project were included and three new markets with no previous CBD exposure were also included. This mixed sample allowed a quasi experimental design to the sub-project which allowed a couple of proposition built around the 4-stage framework to be tested.

The markets with earlier exposure to CBD promotion of RH and FP were likely to make more progress in the promotion of DP and HIV prevention than those with no such experience. And the proportion making a tangible decision indicative of behaviour change such as proceeding to HIV test was likely to be higher in the CBD exposed markets.

The baseline survey of knowledge, attitude and practices relating to HIV/AIDS provided the benchmark indicators which allowed the quantitative changes taking place during the period of intervention to be measured. At the end of the project a sample transept survey of market population and in-depth interviews with market agents yielded further information on the direction of changes in knowledge, attitudes and practices.

Association of LGA/PHC staffers with project markets

With the emphasis of the sub-project on the extent of behaviour change taking place, it was decided that there should be provision for referral PHC in the LGA within which the markets are located. Consequently, a group of midwife/nurses working within those facilities were approached to take part in the sub-project programmes so as to provide the needed backup to the clients to be referred from the markets.

Attainment of goals through selected strategies

For the market-based component of the programmes, the set goals were met in the following areas:
   a) Training of market agents operating in each market;
   b) The organizing of regular open forum market events;
   c) Conduct of monthly review meetings with the agents/cadres;
   d) Regular monitoring of counselling and referral of clients to associated LGA/PHC; and
   e) At the end of intervention, the conduct of the post-intervention evaluation formed the basis of the validation of the applicability of the 4-stage framework to the MARPs in market places.

In the case of the health providers based in the LGA/PHCs the set goals were also in the areas of project take-off training, provision for documentation of project related referrals, participation in monthly market project activities and review of progress and the conduct of the post-evaluation of the facility based aspect of the project.

Training of Market Agents and LGA/CBD staff

Six market associations and LGA/CBD staff in five LGA's were contacted and mobilized for HIV prevention. Baseline surveys were conducted in all six markets and the findings fed into the training curricula for market agents and the LGA/CBD staff respectively. Five of the six markets went on to nominate about 43 agents from their members. They were then trained in DP and HIV/AIDS counselling and service delivery. A total of 12 LGA/CBD staff was also trained in DP/HIV counselling and service delivery.

The occasion of the training allowed the trainees to make contributions to the content and development of IEC materials that were subsequently produced and distributed within and outside the markets. The MIS adopted for market agents took account of the limited literacy and resulted in a simple pictogram that allowed an accurate tally system of the counselling activities of the agents to be maintained.

Market events

Between the training and the end of project activities in August 2002, the agents within each market with the support of the executive boards of the market associations organized monthly market outreach events. ARFH and the LGA/CBD staff gave technical assistance to the agents. Seven monthly events were conducted in each market. The series allowed a systematic selection of IEC materials, topics of discussion and generation of questions and answer sessions built around the respective stages of behaviour changes at each event. This allowed the audience to be taken through the 4-stage framework of behaviour change.

For example, the initial stage of creating awareness of the urgency and reality of the advent of HIV/AIDS in the country and in Oyo state benefited from the selection of video clips which demonstrated graphically the devastation that STIs can cause and the link between STIs and HIV infection. So effective were the video that the first event was generally enough to awaken the attention and concern of the audience to the potential danger posed by the epidemic. Periodically, participants at subsequent events refer to the impression that the clips made upon them. The end of project survey also showed up the video clips as creating the most lasting impression on viewers.

Encouraging people to make competent self risk assessment of the dangers of HIV infection in their own personal lives required more time and a mix of IEC channels. A simple question and anonymous answer session drew attention to the links between life styles and risk of HIV infection. Those who identify one or more risk items were encouraged to reflect on the complications that sexual networking could make to their casual sexual contacts. The degree of extra-marital affairs tolerated by society also raised the stakes for women in particular. Simple drama sketches were also employed to highlight the association of events that conspire to make a simple business trip to a neighbouring country into an unintended casual sexual adventure. So effective were the drama sketches that the content analysis was often occasions for further clarification of the risks attending to the business life styles.

A third component in the second health belief stage aimed at effective risk assessment was the time devoted to questions and answer sessions that addressed some of the concerns people had about their earlier risk taking or about myths surrounding the effectiveness of their own personal prophylactic strategies. In all, by the end of the third monthly event, there was a greater awareness of the vulnerability of all persons regarding the risk of HIV infection.

The remaining two stages of 4-stage framework – that of acquiring knowledge for risk reduction or total elimination of some risks; and the self efficacy needed to put knowledge into practice – raised other issues relating to the selection of IEC material suited to each stage of behaviour change that had the potential to make a difference in the minds of the audience.

Conventional approach to behaviour change communication based on posters, handbills and periodic health talks appeared to be effective in providing the population with the necessary knowledge base. But the process of acquisition of information was enhanced by the technical assistance that the LGA/CBD staffers provided to the open forum and by the tailoring of IEC distribution to each stage of the behaviour change modification. This was the conclusion reached by the systematic observation of open forum sessions for the first two stages of the 4-stage framework.

However, it was with the fourth and final stage that the problems relating to putting knowledge to practice in changing behaviour arose. The motivation to make behaviour change, lack of resources to put knowledge into practice and the negative influence of others on pattern of behaviour led the audiences at the series of event to identifying the fact that inequities existing between men and women, rich and poor, old and young and the powerful and defenceless complicate sexual negotiation and decision making.

In all of the open forum discussions relating to self-efficacy, it was repeatedly stressed that those in powerful positions have a moral obligation to change their pattern of behaviour, if not out of consideration for others, at least for their own self-preservation. However, a culture of pervading moral laxity was seen as the major disincentive to maintaining high safe sexual standards.

In as much as each market event was arranged around the core of market association, agents and the transient market population, some continuity was established between the monthly events. Ideas could be followed through from one event to the other. The regulars at each event number about 50 in each market. The transient audience averaged 200. In effect, the number reached in each market was close to two thousand. One other validation of these estimates was the quantity of IEC materials distributed.

Monthly review meetings

Monthly meetings of agents from all five markets allowed the review of lessons learnt at previous events and the smooth planning of subsequent events. The meetings also gave the agents a sense of ownership and directing the affairs of the programme. It was at these meetings that issues considered peculiar to each market were identified and decisions taken as to how they should influence the conduct of events.

Regular counselling and referral activities

In between monthly events and review meetings, the real tasks performed by each agent consisted of one-on-one counselling, talking to groups and referring contacts to clinics if they needed further clarification on dual protection or wish to pursue the adoption of dual protection in their sexual life. Some male condoms were distributed but this was supplementary to those that were readily available in the open market. The idea of distributing female condoms through the agents was shelved when it was realized that the pelvic models needed for competent counselling of client on use of female condoms were not obtainable within the short life span of the sub-project.

On average each agent talked to 100 on dual protection and related AIDS prevention issues in a month. There was no significant difference between the male and female agents, the agents combined market based activities with those carried out elsewhere in other cultural settings such as in churches and mosques. The number of IEC materials distributed in personal encounters averaged 500 over the life of the sub-project. This was in addition to the distribution of IEC materials during open forum market advocacy events. The accuracy of estimates was made possible by the ease with which the pictograms were completed, the monthly collection of the statistics. The agents were also advised on how to improve the coverage of their activities by extending it beyond the confines of the market into their social networks. The participation of the LGA/CBD staff at the events, monthly meetings and periodic visits to agents also contributed to the high level of adherence to the documentation.

Increasing the chances of success

In summary, the major components of the successful attainment of the goals of the sub-project were:

- Creating an environment of ownership by allowing the agents to emerge from and function within the framework of the market democratic structures. The executive members of market associations saw themselves as hosting the events and the agents saw themselves as functioning on behalf of all members. In effect, the programme did not build up new lines of communication around the agents. This encouraged each of the five markets to think up ways of sustaining the activities beyond the life of the project. ARFH gave the assurance that their efforts in this direction will receive the technical support of the organisation whenever it was asked to make such inputs.

· Allowing an open forum at regular market events demystified the activities of the agents and gave other stall owners a stake in the outcome of the programme. The non-agents saw the agents, therefore, as agents of welcome innovation rather than agents of intrusive/disruptive change.

· The nature of protracted bargaining characteristic of Yoruba selling and buying is a form of social interaction. This made agent-client interactions on dual protection counselling compatible with the norms of the market place. Private counselling of clients under these conditions did not appear intrusive. For the more experienced agents it was seen as a social obligation to their friends, family and casual clients that they exchange views on current affairs of which the HIV/AIDS epidemic was the most compelling.

Discussions on market agents

Some of the market agents came to the programme with the head start of participating in the CBD programmes in the 1980s. This was beneficial to the implementation of the programme. It was amazing that in spite of their knowledge of family planning objectives, they were as responsive to the issues of dual protection promotion as other groups involved in similar enterprise. The challenged posed by AIDS prevention was found by them to be as relevant as for those with no previous CBD experience.

An impression emerged over the life of the project which made the agents more open in discussing the extent of sexual risk taking going on within their respective trading profession. The issue of sex for services that has influenced the spread of HIV/AIDS in other parts of Africa was present in the marketing situation. The discussion of the drama sketches which formed a staple of monthly open market events often revealed some of the mechanisms of the sexual risk-taking that went on in the markets.

Conclusion to market agent sub-project

The market sub-project turned out to be the most interactive platform of all of the sub-projects. The market-events allowed the participation of a cross-section of the population in a way not possible in other venues. It was in this context that some of the startling revelations about paedophilia in Yoruba society were made. Pre-teen children were not only sexually active within their age groups but in contact with adults. There was no apparent link between the AIDS epidemic and the advent of paedophilia as was the case in some other societies/countries where a search for non-infected children fuelled the phenomenon (Earl-Taylor, 2002).

The reservoir of skills and goodwill accumulated in the market agent programme was later put to use in reaching other parts of Oyo State and in the development of more ambitious biomedical cum biosocial intervention within the market agent population in form of HIV surveillance sub project which forms the topic of the next chapter.
The market agent sub-project has further reinforced the credibility of the market based CBD approach. The area of policy impact was the potential that existed to incorporate the market agents into a Local Government level management of Primary Health Care.

INVOLVING PRIVATE HEALTH SECTOR IN PROMOTING DUAL PROTECTION

Introduction

Most health sector analysts agree that the private health sector accounts for nearly two-thirds of reproductive health services; that the sector was made more attractive to clients by their physical and cultural closeness to their clients; that the profit motive in the private sector make the staff more accountable than in the public sector; and that the professional medical and other health providers association provide a platform for standard setting. Consequently, the project identified general practice facilities providing reproductive health services as a viable platform for the promotion of dual protection and the associated behaviour change.

The DP approach was based on the training of health providers in counselling skills with which to systematically counsel both male and female clients on the prevailing HIV/AIDS epidemic. They were also to explain the associated risks people face in their current sexual behaviour and practices. The need for the clients to make appropriate sexual behaviour modification and have the power to make appropriate choices was also to be stressed. The project integrated the approach into general practice through a programme of training of health providers on HIV/AIDS Basic, sexual risk assessment, HIV counselling, and referral of clients to STI and HIV testing facilities. In addition, four periodic updates were given the doctors/proprietors of the private medical health facilities.

After the training the proprietors and staff of the facilities were provided with IEC materials and technical assistance as well as MIS forms with which they documented their activities on the project. They were also encouraged to monitor their own performances so that the project interventions could be sustained after the project ended. Throughout, various forms of continuous advocacy were carried out as a means of sustaining general community interest in dual protection and in the opportunities offered by health providers within the private medical health facilities. The project outcome was a higher level of contribution of general medical practice to the improvement of reproductive and sexual health in the population.

Choice of strategies for the attainment of DP/BCC goals

In retrospect, the various strategies played different roles in the acceptability of the project interventions in the different MARPS and by the individual members of each population. For example the selection of facilities was preceded by a baseline survey of the human and material resources and the range of services provided in about 80 private health facilities within Ibadan metropolis that met the preliminary criterion that they provided some reproductive health services to the public. The survey and the dissemination of the results among the proprietors of the facilities assured them of the objectivity of the project and its methods.

The training for DP providers faced the challenge of the differences in educational and professional skills that they bring to the task. An added complication was that proprietors had different standards in the quality of staff they hire in their respective facilities. The training programme took account of this issue by tailoring the content, methods and duration of training to the capacities of the providers. The emphasis was on enhancing the counselling and peer education skills at all levels. The Community Health Extension Workers (CHEWs) and auxiliaries were given extra attention since they were usually the first point of contact for clients coming to the facilities.

At the end of the selection process, a total of 43 private health sector facilities were involved in the project. Over 50 nurses, midwives and auxiliaries were trained in DP counselling, and related services. 23 physicians participated in four bi-monthly updates at which they were made aware of the latest information regarding issues such as VCT, ART, PMTCT and universal precautions relating to HIV/AIDS prevention in the work place.

In terms of performance, the CHEWs and auxiliaries were predominantly responsible for the introductory peer education and general health talks while the nurses and midwives gave additional in depth information and counselling on AIDS prevention strategies appropriate to the circumstances of each client. The arrangement for the processing of clients also provided an opportunity to stage the behaviour change as clients moved from provider to provider. The general health talks formed the basis of awareness creation. The nurses and midwives assisted the process of personal risk assessment and provision of information for risk reduction. Ultimately, the clients took responsibility for putting the new knowledge gained into practice, that is, to the extent to which they had the negotiating skills and power to effect necessary behaviour modification and changes with the full cooperation of their sexual partners.

The differences in tasks were reflected in the number of clients counselled by both cadres. On average, the auxiliaries did twice as much counselling as the nurse/midwives. In addition, because the auxiliaries were socially and culturally closer to the clients they served, information from them were well received by the clients. It was also easier for them, within their social cycles, to extend their peer education activities beyond the health facility setting. To some of them, the peer education skill was an added value that empowered them to function outside the narrow framework of their official facility functions.

The faith-based organisations to which these auxiliaries belonged were the secondary targets of their peer education activities. Some of the nurse/midwives also took on additional community based peer education and counselling responsibilities, but to a lesser extent than their younger and junior colleagues who had relatively less responsibilities in health facilities. The motivation to gain relevance and prestige in their respective communities was apparently higher among these auxiliaries and CHEWs than among the nurse/midwives.

The basic MIS employed in the private sector health facilities was similar to the one used during the in-school project. The review of the MIS in monthly meetings was also a way of assuring that documentation of DP/BCC peer education and counselling activities in the respective facilities was complete and accurate. The monthly meetings also served the occasion for discussing any problems and solutions found in different facilities during the project implementation.

After the take-off 5-day comprehensive training, the 28 providers with accurate MIS records had each counselled an average of 100 clients in one-on-one interaction every month for the 10 months of intervention. In effect, a total of 28,000 individuals were involved in such personalized counselling sessions. The group counselling sessions involved an average of 20 clients gathered together within the health facilities. But during the outreach activities outside the clinics, the averages rose to over a hundred. The number of persons reached in these group sessions totalled 25,000.

Increasing the chances of success

There were three elements of the private health sector involvement in promoting DP that contributed to the measure of success achieved. They were a) the involvement of doctors in regular updates which kept up their interest and support for the programme; b) the development of jointly organized community outreach programmes which bring a number of clinics together in collaboration rather than in competition; and c) the exceptional commitment of some facilities to the project.

a) Doctors' update as advocacy

In most of the clinics, the doctors did not engage in counselling sessions. However, some were occasionally responsible for "one-on-one" further counselling of clients during consultation. Some doctors also delivered the health talks during community outreach, bringing their reputation and prestige to bear on the seriousness of purpose. The doctors also contributed to successful project implementation by accommodating the additional time that their staff devoted to clients in promoting DP. A further measure of their commitment to AIDS prevention took the form of their regular attendance at the updates on various aspects of the control and management of the epidemic.

Five such updates were conducted during the project period. The method for each update included the use of multi-media material available on published CDs with such topics as:

- "DISCOVERY: An interactive investigation of HIV and AIDS" (GlaxoWellcome);
- "Highlights from the 7th Conference on Retroviruses and Opportunistic Infections" (HRSA TRI);
- "Highlights from the XIII International AIDS Conference, Durban, South Africa" (HRSA TRI); and
- "Economics in HIV/AIDS planning: Getting priorities right" (UNAIDS).

The content of the multimedia CDs stimulated lively discussions of clinical experiences of the participating doctors. To expand the scope of discussions, most sessions had a social scientist (the principal investigator) acting as facilitator.

b) Cooperative approach to health facilities' outreach into the community

Another devise that facilitated the smooth implementation of the programme was the formation of participating clinics in each Local Government Area into informal co-sponsors of joint outreach activities in their neighbourhood. This arrangement created a network of potential support clinics for the control and management of HIV/AIDS. Attention was turned away from the special skills and focus of each clinic, to addressing the pressing needs of the community in area of AIDS prevention. The outcome was an increase in the referral between clinics and a sharing of resources in addressing occasional emergencies.

c) Other Predictors of commitment

Over and above the updates and the outreach programmes, there were other circumstances of each health facility that encouraged their active involvement in AIDS prevention through the promotion of DP. The first factor was the familiarity of the doctors with HIV/AIDS cases prior to the project implementation. The very few doctors who saw cases but were not particularly enthused with clinical management of HIV/AIDS turned out to be very supportive of DP programmes. The measure of that support took the form of investing in pelvic models with which to deliver female condoms even when it was clear that there was no way that FCs could be distributed other than at highly subsidized prices.

Another indicator of commitment was linked to the structure of facility management. Clinics in which a husband and wife medical team were in charge were likely to be more committed to AIDS prevention activities and making necessary resource inputs into DP promotion than clinics where there was a sole male health professional in charge.

Coping with Peculiarities

A number of operational problems arose during the project implementation. These problems relate to a) inequalities in the human and resource capacities of the facilities; b) differences in the scope of services provided in each facility; and c) preferences of proprietors about possible involvement in the clinical management of AIDS cases.

a) Varying capacities of facilities

The baseline survey of private health facilities partly prepared project staff for the problem of uneven performance that was to arise from differences in the human and material resources which were available in each clinic. Consequently, the focus of training was to make each cadre of provider as well equipped as possible in coping with the responsibilities attached to the systematic promotion of DP. A further complication was that the number of staff available in a clinic was not always related to the number of clients. In effect, the workload of staff varied significantly from facility to facility. The result of these differences was to produce a situation in which the level of performance on DP promotion equally varied. The regular progress review meetings allowed providers to share tips on tactics for improving the situation.

b) Differences in scope of services

Another feature of the baseline differences between facilities was the scope of services each provided their clients. Some of the larger facilities, by the range and depth of services provided attracted a larger patronage than others. The more the focus of facilities on reproductive health per se, the easier it was for them to integrate the promotion of DP in their services. Other facilities with a focus on general health care services found it more difficult to set the space and time apart to be able to make a systematic effort at promoting DP.

c) Preferences of proprietors about HIV/AIDS case management

Partly in response to the pattern of services they had on ground, a number of facilities saw their primary role as raising awareness about the need for DP. The actual distribution of condoms or programmes of voluntary counselling and testing were considered as out of the scope of their interest. For others, the following up of clients tested for STIs and HIV demanded more staff time and resources than they could spare. A few had considered the economic impact of care and support for AIDS cases on their practices as unacceptable. The positions of such doctors and proprietors were repeated topic of discussions at the updates. It is fair to add that some changed their positions, becoming more involved in HIV/AIDS prevention and management.

Discussion of the General Practice DP/BCC project

The major surprise of the General Practice DP/BCC sub-project which reflected on the power of the adopted 4-stage framework BCC model was the dramatic change in the attitude of doctors to the whole issue of HIV/AIDS prevention. It was initially difficult to gain their attention and enthusiasm about direct involvement in project activities, since most did not do counselling of patients in any consistent sense of that activity. However, the more they were given the background information about developments in the control and management of HIV/AIDS, the more their interest increased. Towards the end of the project, their professional association showed great interest in the updates organized. Some doctors whose clinics were not in the sub-project took part in updates. ARFH has since the conclusion of the intervention been able to draw paying doctors to some other updates on issues of interest to them. Participating doctors also used their standing in the Association of General and Private Medical Practitioners of Nigeria (AGPMPN), Oyo State chapter by inserting some updates into the monthly discussions of the state-wide Association.

Conclusion to General Practice DP/BCC project

The feasibility of involving private sector facilities in the promotion of dual protection has been demonstrated. Consistent counselling and referral of clients for more information on dual protection practices and services were introduced in the 43 clinics. In three of them, acquisition of pelvic models has allowed the distribution of a limited amount of female condoms. Between them, the three were able to distribute a monthly average of 40 female condoms to the handful of clients on their books.

Since the promotion of dual protection was the first attempt for some of them to systematically deliver family planning services, it will take some time to discover what impact the female condom can have in private health facilities. From what we know from other ARFH dual protection activities in family planning settings, the acceptability of female condom was reasonable. The FC was convenient for some clients as a stand-alone method. But the majority of family planning clients found the convenience of making female condoms a combined method with their existing contraceptive more attractive.

DETAILS OF AIDS PREVENTION PROGRAMMES

The common components of three MARPS HIV prevention projects on which some additional comments are worth making are a) the Training of peers and providers; b) Development and distribution of IEC materials and a Behaviour Change Communication model based on multimedia IEC strategy; and c) The policy impact of the series of AIDS prevention programmes.

Training of peer educators, counsellors, market agents and health providers

The challenge of the training programme was to device suitable training curriculum for the different categories of peer educators and health providers in the variety of platforms in which they functioned. In all, there were 8 different curriculum and contents developed for the respective cadres on the projects:
1. In-school peer educators curriculum
2. Teacher sexual health counsellors curriculum
3. Out of school youth and adult peer educators curriculum
4. Youth friendly PHC clinic staff curriculum
5. Market based DP peer educators curriculum
6. Private health facility health providers (nurses and midwives) curriculum
7. Private health facility auxiliary staff (CHEW and others) curriculum and
8. Updates for doctors

In the end, ARFH drew on its experiences on developing curricula for various programmes in designing appropriate content for each of the training exercises. An evaluation of the set of trainings found that the training objectives were effectively met. The specific issues involved in each of the training for each of the three sub-projects were as follows:

Training of peer educators and school counsellors
The position of peer educators in schools was somewhat different from those of out-of-school youths, some of whom were in sub-ordinate position to trade masters and other category of adults to whom they deferred in matters of earning a living or in their living arrangements. The literacy levels between the two groups did not differ significantly since some literacy was a precondition for being able to cope with the responsibilities of the peer educator which included the distribution of IEC materials and in explaining IEC contents to others as well as keeping a simple record of their activities. In the end, belonging to the same age cohort and potentially exposed to the same life styles were bases for adopting broadly similar contents for the training of both groups of peer educators.

The teachers were selected as sexual health counsellors on the basis of their aptitude or existing responsibilities in shaping adolescent character in their respective schools. They therefore brought to the training a higher knowledge base about handling youths even if their AIDS prevention knowledge base was low. In effect, the emphasis in the training of the teachers was on equipping them with counselling skills.

Training of market agents as peer educators

In devising the training curriculum for market agents, some of the basic skills which they had were built upon. Such skills include negotiating sales, presenting clients with choices on the basis of price and other considerations and keeping records of their activities. In addition, account was taken of the fact that some came to the project with experiences in community or market based distribution of contraceptives in the late 1980's. On the down side, a few had no previous exposure to CBD programmes. Some were not articulate in English but were fully literate in the local language – Yoruba. This one aspect of their composition made the conduct of the training in Yoruba a necessity. In all the five participating markets both sexes were equally represented in the selection of agents that was made at the respective market association meetings according to the profiles of eligible agents provided to them by ARFH.

One outstanding quality of the people selected as market agents was their responsiveness to the idea of a culture sensitive 4-stage framework health belief model with which they and their clients could achieve the behaviour change needed to adequately slow the spread of HIV/AIDS in Oyo State. An elaboration of the four stages into a schema for carrying out a series of market outreach monthly events over a period of 9 to 10 months produced a remarkable programme of behaviour change communication within this and other sub-projects. Consequently, the minimum of 6 outreach events was rescheduled to allow for another two sessions so that the gains of the BCC can be consolidated.

Training of health providers

Since the central objective of the DP in GP programme was to systematically provide clients with DP counselling, referral and, where possible, barrier methods, the selection of health providers to be trained was guided by the need to train at least two individuals from each of the participating clinics. This arrangement made provision for the shift duty system subsisting in the health services and made allowance for the rapid turnover of staff in the private health sector. Going to training increases the mobility of health providers whose chances of moving to larger practices improved on the strength of the new skills acquired in such trainings.

The turn-over of staff of the facilities during the life of the project was amazingly low and may have been an outcome of the network of clinics encouraged by the project in contrast to the rivalries created by competing private health practices.

IEC FOR BEHAVIOUR CHANGE – TRIBUNE CARTOON SERIES

The components of the behaviour change communication in each of the sub-projects were firmly rooted in the principles of maximizing group activities, employing a multimedia approach and innovating in the facilitation of activities. Development of simple record keeping instrument allowed a prompt analysis of the progress each change agent was making.

To complement the activities among the ARPS, a cartoon series corresponding to the different stages of the 4-stage framework was run in The Tribune newspaper over a period of 20 weeks.

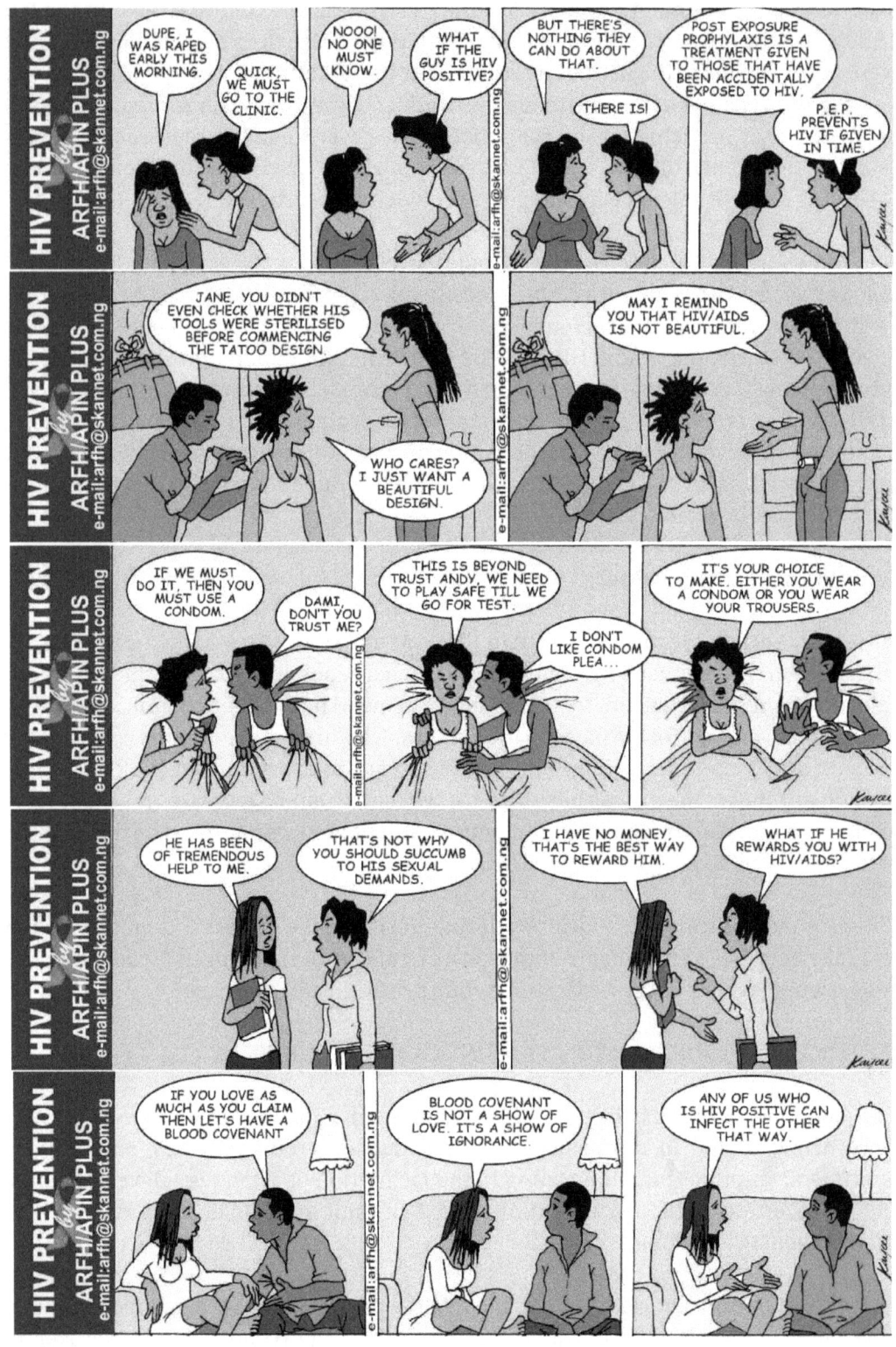

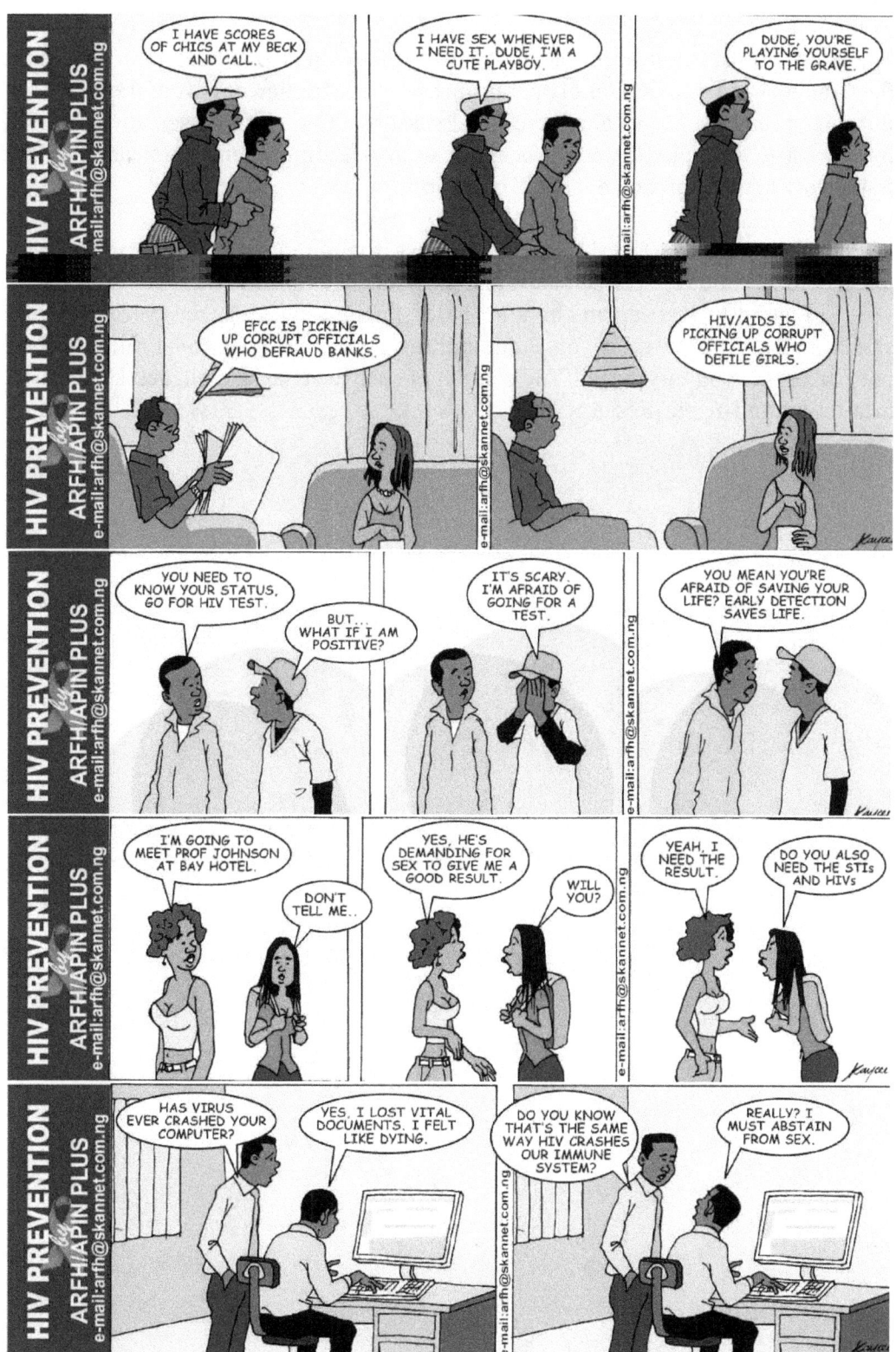

CONCLUSION

The promotion of HIV prevention among ARPS provided an opportunity to appreciate the strengths and weaknesses of operating the 4-stage framework in different settings. But the strengths outweighed the weaknesses. The cultural sensitivity of the framework made it possible for target populations to comprehend the structure of the framework in terms of their own local perception of issues.

Those who were not very literate could base their understanding largely on the interpersonal contacts between them and the peer educators or with other people who were prepared to step down the knowledge to them with spoken words. Drama sketches are familiar mode of communicating ideas in traditional societies and particularly among the Yoruba. The content of such sketches are aligned closely with local drama and movie products.

CHAPTER 8
HIV SURVEILLANCE
IN IBADAN AND OGBOMOSO MARKETS

INTRODUCTION

At the end of the promotion of behaviour change in Ibadan markets, among in- and out-of-school youth and in Private Health Facilities between 2001 and 2002, the validity of the 4-stage framework was well established. One of the main lessons learnt from those three projects was the feasibility of increasing knowledge and effecting some behavioural changes in the different demographic and social groups. In addition, the improved understanding and appreciation of HIV prevention by those who participated in project activities were passed on to others within and outside the locations of study. Peer educators in the markets voluntarily reached out to members of the community and so did the PEs in private health facilities and in schools.

Some increase in condom use provided a quantitative indicator of behaviour change. Evaluation of interventions among the target groups showed significant closing of the gap between stages 2 and 3 of the 4-stage framework, on the one hand, and stage 4 on the other. Personal vulnerability was recognized by participants, and information on where, how and when to seek prophylactic services and treatment of infections was well comprehended. However it was on the basis of effective exposure to negotiation of sexual interactions that people were able to change their risky behaviour for the adoption of safer sex practices (Kippax et. al., 1997).

But access to VCT services was required if people were to embrace regular counselling and testing as a non sexual prophylactic or infection management strategy. As a way of redressing this limitation of the first set of interventions, a collaborative intervention combining the social science based 4-stage framework methodologies with a biomedical programme of HIV surveillance was the logical next step. This phase of the study was implemented jointly by the Association of Reproductive and Family Health (ARFH) and the Department of Virology, UCH, Ibadan over the 24-month period from 2003 to 2005 to test a number of propositions borne out of the earlier lessons learnt. Those propositions include the following:

a. The intensity and quality of multimedia BCC programmes determine the extent to which the target populations gain in-depth understanding of issues, internalize the messages and make an effort to alter undesirable practices.

b. Given the life style of the market population, sustaining interest in a multi-round VCT programme required detailed preparation. The actual biomedical intervention was introduced on the back of a carefully planned biosocial programme which involved advocacy to opinion leaders, formative research, baseline studies, and a well thought out dissemination of the results to the surveyed population. This was followed by the selection and in-depth training of interested peer educator volunteers from the population who later educated the network of individuals and groups within and outside the market system who need access to the HIV treatment and support services.

c. That the indicators of a breakthrough in the combined biosocial/biomedical VCT programme will include the ease with which set recruitment targets are met, the proportions of people obtaining their results and the proportion proceeding to subsequent rounds of the programme.

d. That the social networks built around the VCT programme will become a potent agent for creating the culture of VCT as a viable HIV/AIDS prevention and management option not only in the target populations but in the wider community.

It should be noted that the third proposition is based on the recognition that some of the changes that people made in response to the biosocial interventions such as reduction of partners and use of condom in sexual activities do not lend themselves to direct observation. In contrast the act of taking a VCT and receiving the results and acting on referral activities or the repetition of the HIV test in subsequent round of tests is concrete evidence of the attainment of the stage 4 of the 4-stage framework. It is also apparent that such a level of commitment to change carries greater emotional and pragmatic attitudes to self preservation. Consequently, the planning, implementation and evaluation of the HIV project is the focus of this chapter so that its role in the further development of the 4-stage framework can be understood.

Research design 2 and 2 Control and Intervention Markets
In an attempt to improve the validity of the 4-stage framework, the HIV surveillance project was extended from Ibadan where most of the previous projects had taken place to include Ogbomoso. This extension was also in recognition of the higher HIV prevalence rates for the northern parts of Oyo State reported in the sentinel survey. In addition, the market places were adjudged the most appropriate for the HIV surveillance study since they allowed some assurance of continued contacts for VCT and for the follow up of volunteers.

Two markets in each town were designated as the intervention markets and two markets were designated as the control markets so as to allow for the testing of the propositions. In the intervention markets, the full 4-stage framework and laboratory services for the four rounds of 6-montly testing, notification, referral and follow up were carried out. In contrast, only the 4-stage framework behaviour promotional activities were carried out in the control markets without the VCT services.

With this experimental design, all the eight markets were exposed to the benefits of the behaviour change model and where applicable were referred to VCT services in Ogbomoso and Ibadan. The design also allowed the continued validation of the 4-

stage framework on its own or in combination with the provision of VCT services. The 8 markets with their location and experimental statuses were as follows: Aaradaa and Oja Titun markets were the two intervention markets in Ogbomoso whilst Oja Oba was the control market. In Ibadan, Anajere and Owode Academy markets were the two intervention markets whilst Mokola and Bodija markets were the control markets. Strategies for HIV Surveillance in Ibadan and Ogbomoso markets

In recognition of the greater sensitivity of delivering VCT services in addition to the biosocial strategies employed in the earlier projects, a number of inter-related strategies were devised for the surveillance. Although some of the elements of the strategies had been described in earlier chapters, the range of strategies employed on the surveillance is described briefly in this chapter so that a replication of such a project can be attempted elsewhere. The peculiar circumstances introduced into project implementation by the nature of the combined biosocial and biomedical activities will also be clarified.

The strategies were:
1. The formation and training of a joint UCH/ARFH project team in research methodology and ethics which was responsible for all programmes and activities in the field;
2. The conduct of an energetic advocacy to the palace, local government areas in which markets are located, the market leadership and the separate trade groups in those markets, and to proprietors of private medical health facilities that were already involved in HIV screening and referral;
3. The mobilization of the general market in open forums as basis of project take off and the conduct of the baseline KABP survey of population samples drawn from the markets followed by a quick dissemination of findings to the market open forum; leading to
4. The Recruitment, Training and Deployment of volunteer peer educators from the market open forums and from trade groups, and of health counsellors nominated from private health facilities;
5. The mobilization of materials and resources (laboratory equipment, test kits, counselling rooms, registers etc) for on the spot testing and notification of results
6. The VCT and notification sessions;
7. The conduct of ten monthly sessions of BCC interventions in open forums in both experimental and control markets so the behaviour modification and change benefits of the project is not denied to the control markets.
8. The review of progress made by subgroups of the project participants – counsellors from private health facilities, general market population, all trained PE volunteers, all who volunteered for multi-round HIV tests and results;

STRATEGY DESCRIPTIONS

The elaboration of the methodology and short term outcomes of these strategies form the central material for this chapter. Each is described below with attention paid to the appropriateness of the strategy, the benefits and challenges of its implementation and the extent to which it contributed to the overall goal of encouraging and sustaining changes in risky behaviour and taking necessary precautions and actions that enhance the chances of preventing or surviving HIV infection.

1. **The formation and training of a joint UCH/ARFH project team in research methodology and ethics which was responsible for all programmes and activities in the field**

In any joint project, and especially in multi-disciplinary one, making sure that field staff know their roles and how those fit into other roles, is important to smooth operations and multi-tasking by members of the team. A joint team made up of laboratory scientists, counsellors, data clerks and sociologists and virologists was formed at the start of the project. They went through a 10-day training on research methodology, research ethics and role playing of activities to be carried out in the field. They were also able to work out those tasks for which there could be opportunities to be polyvalent so as to reduce the volunteers' waiting time.

The training was also able to break the ice between a team made up of people with difference in education, discipline and background so that an easy working relationship was forged before the project implementation began.

2. **The conduct of an energetic advocacy to the palace, local government areas in which markets are located, the market leadership and the separate trade groups in those markets, and to proprietors of private medical health facilities that were already involved in HIV screening and referral**

Advocacy was conducted to Ogbomoso starting at the highest level at the Palace of Soun down to the leaders of the Intervention and control markets. The project leader was very instrumental in the process, being a native of the town. The advocacy in Ibadan did not require the same effort as there were ongoing projects on HIV prevention in the selected markets. Consequently, the intervention was built on the existing lines of communication and approval procedures.

The market leaders gave their approval after consulting with the various market trade unions. In addition, the project team was given an opportunity to go over the details of what was to happen on the project, the eligibility for participation and the conditions of participating. At the end of the process of consultation, the number of participants to attend the peer counselling training, the timing of training and the time table for the process of VCT, and the arrangement for the notification of results and referral to UCH for those testing positive were agreed. In the control markets the timing of the 4-stage framework promotional activities were agreed so that the disruption of trading activities was kept to a minimum whilst the conduct of project intervention was allowed all the time needed for its effectiveness and replication of procedures which had been established in earlier projects.

3. **The mobilization of the general market in open forums as basis of project take off and the conduct of the baseline KABP survey and dissemination of results**

In an attempt to bring the general market population into the early stages of the project implementation, the open forum strategy was adopted. Over two successive market days, the project team interacted with the market population at the venue of their open forum meetings. It was at these interactions that the purpose and plans for the project was presented and the support of the market was obtained.

The plans included the conduct of a sample survey in the four markets and the subsequent dissemination of the results. The dissemination forum then formed the basis of implementing the recruitment, training and deployment of volunteer peer educators.

4. **The Recruitment, Training and Deployment of volunteer peer educators from the market open forums and from trade groups, and health counsellors nominated from private health facilities**

Formal training allowed time for raising awareness of the epidemic and of the opportunities for HIV prevention. It allowed the inculcating of new values, passing on new skills and developing confidence in the management of health related behaviour by participants. The second strategy of project team keeping regular contacts with volunteers allowed their learning to be reinforced and the problems arising from changing their behaviour to be resolved through experience sharing among the project participants and exchange of tips on solving problems during the monthly review meetings held among different groups in the markets.

Three sets of training were conducted: The volunteers in the market had a tailor made training aimed at encouraging them along the lines of the 4-stage framework. Staff of the private health facilities who had been involved in some limited VCT was also trained so that their counselling and referral systems will function along the latest protocol available and so that they can work with the project in such a way as to increase its multiplier effect. The proprietors of the private health facilities were also involved in a programme of knowledge update of the type that took place in Ibadan under the outreach programme to the AGMPN (see chapter 7).

Peer educator training
The purpose of training, the required attendance level and benefits of the training to

participants were explained at general market place planning meetings. The volunteers had to be able to find the time for both the training and for the follow up responsibilities of counselling others about HIV prevention, distribution of IEC materials and the keeping of a basic record of their activities. The primary school education that most of them had was enough for these tasks.

Take off training for volunteers

The take off training for 150 volunteers from the pair of markets in each town took place over a period of 10 days. Because they had been involved in the planning of the training, they were able to plan the time-table around their daily activities and, in Ogbomoso, around the Muslim fasting period which was going on at the same time.

The content was built around the 4 stages of the behaviour change model. Formal information about the state of the HIV epidemic in Nigeria and in Oyo State formed the basic information for the rest of the content. The awareness creation stage made use of formal lectures on the nature of the epidemic, the transmission, incubation, progression and stages of infection, and emergence of full blown AIDS. The presentation was supplemented with graphic video clips from the "Silent Epidemic" a feature film which, though dated, was factual and very graphic and effective in communication the seriousness of some of the consequences of infections of STDs and HIV. Additional learning materials were in the form of commentaries from the facilitators about the causes and spread of the epidemic. Advantage was also taken of the enthusiasm of volunteers for local drama sketches to illustrate some of the situations and settings surrounding unsafe sex practices and the exposure to the risk of infection. All discussions were all in the Yoruba language understood by all the peer education volunteers.

Unlike conventional printed IEC Materials the interpretation of which presented some people with challenges (Bankole, 1982), the video material and the interactive viewing in a training situation made the intent and message explicit. As pointed elsewhere in the book (Chapter 4), the raw images in the film "The Silent Epidemic" confronted trainees with an inescapable urgency and seriousness of the epidemic and of the physical and social impact of STIs including HIV/AIDS.

At subsequent sessions in the 10-day training, attention and materials shifted to the other stages of the 4-stage framework. The stage of self risk assessment was relatively easy as it was built around discussion of sexual experiences of participants and their analysis of how safe or not those practices were in the context of their observations and insights into the nature of the epidemic in earlier sessions. It must be added that the market population by their life style are more open and expansive about their sexuality (Adeokun, 1982).

The major revelations at the vulnerability sessions were as follows:
- There was a significant but unavoidable use of sex in trade transactions

especially in the meat trade where a relatively scarce resource was being distributed by men to competing bidders who were predominantly female.

· At the end of the trading day, parts of the market were often empty and cosy enough for transient sexual encounters between traders or between traders and lovers from outside the market.

· There was consensus that the sexual encounters were often unprotected and the proposed use of condom was either not taken seriously by some or the suggestion found to be offensive in that it is based on the assumption that there is suspicion of pre-existing STD or HIV infection in one of the partners. The male partners were mostly not keen on condoms and the female partners consider the proposed use of one an accusation of loose sexual life.

· By all the standard measures of risk factors of HIV infection, the participants realised that they were without exception at risk in one way or the other. Even the most faithful of wives could not guarantee that their husbands were faithful Two-thirds of survey respondents at baseline suggested they either were sure their husbands were cheating or they suspected they were.

· Above all, there was unanimity that given the raised awareness they had gained so far in the opening training sessions, they were committed to staying on the training and eventually participating in the periodic HIV surveillance VCT sessions. The two reasons they gave were that the first test will let them know if they are already infected and as explained in the HIV Basics, do something about the infection. And if they were not infected thank God and watch out for the risk factors of infection in their sexual life.

Depending on the pace of understanding of the training sessions, by the 6th day of the training, attention generally shifted to the third stage which focussed on the acquisition of regular and updated information about the epidemic. For this phase, attention was focused on providing the peer educators with oral and written information on various hospitals and clinics where people can access VCT or obtain information and services about STDs, Family Planning and HIV/AIDS services. General Practitioners were often invited to participate by making presentations to the trainees about the patient flows and procedures in their clinics.

In the general discussion about the usefulness of the information, two reservations were made by the participants. Unlike the free tests that were to be made available on the project in the markets during the two year period, tests were not free in other clinics. The second observation was regret that even their family members will not have access to the project's free test services.

With regards to the fourth stage of the 4-stage framework, the training reverted to the methods of the self risk assessment session by encouraging discussion about the participants' chances of being able to fully implement the prophylactic and other HIV infection risk reduction in their lives. The first step was the feedback to the participants of the findings of the baseline survey of KABP about sexual practices in their communities. The discussion that followed allowed the validation of the findings by opening the aggregate findings through the informal reactions to the findings.

Next attention was turned to the existing power relations between sexual partners in their social cycles. Attention was drawn to the dominant and upper hand males exercised in sexual practices including the refusal to use the male condom. The cultural and social undertones of the male dominance were also discussed. According to the volunteers, males had greater access to resources such as farm produce, cattle and slaughtered meat as well as cash. Society accorded them the greater liberties in sexual matters and socialized women to be nice to their male partners.

When asked what the implications of the power relations will mean for the ability to adjust their sexual practices in favour of risk reduction, the males emphasized the demand that the epidemic will make on male self discipline and greater recognition that the motive for such changes in their sexual practices were most likely going to be in response to their own safety now that they know how lethal the HIV infection can be. The females agreed with the male analysis and pointed out that the cultural norms guiding male female social and sexual interactions were not going to be changed unless spearheaded by male. They added that males had hitherto been indifferent to the social and material costs of inconvenient pregnancies, infections and social stigma that females face.

It was in the context of the apparent gender divide about sexual practices and norms that the volunteers were encouraged to suggest what options were open to either gender to address the challenges of the HIV/AIDS epidemic. In effect, the volunteers led the identification of negotiating options open to women in coping with the unequal power relations. Whilst the women emphasised the role that their new knowledge could play in such negotiation, the men focused on their own fear of the consequences of inaction about risk reduction. In effect, the women planned to rely on their knowledge base to peer educate their partners and effect change in them. In contrast, the men held on the notion of their greater power base but conceded that the prospect of HIV/AIDS in their lives was going to be too costly to be ignored.

At the end of the training, it was agreed that the progress the volunteers made in the communication of their information to others as well as the changes that they made in their sexual and other risk taking will be subject to review in the monthly gatherings which would be organized in each market over the course of the two years. In retrospect, the progress in encouraging the peer educators to be enthusiastic about the project was, in part due to the excellent facilitation. This was acknowledged in the assessment made by the peer educators at the end of each session as well as in the post training evaluation. The other factor of success at the training was the sequence of training materials along the lines of the planned path of behaviour range. It meant that the participants were prepared for the turn of discussion as a logical extension of what they have already learnt and what they think is additional skills and information they need to have so as to address the issues raised in previous stage.

Update for Proprietors of collaborating health facilities

It will be remembered that in the earlier phase of the project, Proprietors of collaborating health facilities in Ibadan (all members of the AGMPN) received updates on both the basic science and direction of HIV research prior to the training of the health workers on counselling and project implementation strategies.

To achieve the same level of understanding of issues and assure the collaboration of the proprietors in Ogbomoso an approach was made to those of them who were known to be involved in the screening for HIV and in the management of infections. The baseline survey of the facilities revealed that the services being given were within the limitations in their knowledge and resources. In addition, there was the impact of the unavoidable profit motive on the quality of their services. Consequently, the test fees were on the high side and certainly a constraint to high uptake. The quality of counselling varied from facility to facility since the counsellors did not have a standard training course. Also, without exception, the facilities did not pay as much attention to ethical issues as was required to avoid some of the clients' anecdotes of breach of confidentiality, sharing patient information with relevant others and in some instances with third parties with the approval of the clients.

Against this situation on the ground, appropriately modified course contents were prepared for the updates. The emphasis was on sharing the most recent information on the national policy, the scientific progress being made in the management of HIV infection, the role that the UCH PEPFAR clinic was playing in the treatment and care of patients as well as introduce them to the notions of behaviour change based on structuring the information shared with patients in the course of their treatment and encouraging all facility clients to embark on behaviour change in response to the HIV/AIDS epidemic.

Because of the dramatic changes in the National HIV/AIDS policy between December 2003 and 2004, the role of the private health facilities changed considerably and there was a greater enthusiasm on their part to collaborate with the HIV surveillance project. Prior to the policy change, the private facilities had a number of options for people testing HIV positive: They could be referred to the Baptist Hospital, they could be asked to source for ARV from Ilorin or they could be referred to the UCH. The cost of ARV at the time was ₦12,000.00 (twelve thousand naira) for a month's supply. But by December 2003, the Federal Government under President Olusegun Obasanjo made HIV test and ARV free. The loss of testing fees in the health facilities was more than made up by the more assured line of referral to UCH PEPFAR clinic and access to free ARV and consistent monitoring and management of patients. For the patients too, the greater assurance of competent treatment and management in Ibadan came at a cost since those living in Ogbomoso had to find the cost of travel for the three-hour journey and lost a day of trade into the bargain.

Training of HIV counsellors from local health facilities

Sixteen HIV/AIDS health counsellors were trained on the project from the two towns. The purpose of their training was to take care of referrals that would be generated from the four experimental and three control project markets. Prior to the training, a recruitment visit was made to Health facilities/ hospitals around the project markets and a total of four health providers were recruited for the training in each town. The Ogbomoso group was made up of one male and three females. The facilities represented at the training were selection on the bases of their close proximity to the project markets in Ogbomoso.

In an attempt to broaden the support base for the market programme and share the unique training model used on the project, the health counsellors were give a 5-day update peer education training programme of the type provided for the market based volunteer peer educators. The outcome was that they were positioned to handle the ongoing HIV prevention counselling needs of their own clients along the lines of the 4-stage framework. In effect, people outside the market could benefit from the referral channels opened up through the market project even if they did not work in the markets.

Because members of this group were already involved in HIV counselling, their reaction to the training content was more aligned with the differences between what they experienced in the health facilities and what contributions the new learning will make to their work. In common with the market peer educators they found the awareness creation materials quite convincing and suggested it should be made more widely available to the general public. They felt that copies could be used in their facilities during the group counselling sessions prior to individual counselling sessions. The health workers acknowledged that some clients continued to have reservations about acknowledging their risk factors when in private health facilities. The health workers also raised the issue of the extended counselling time required for the risk assessment. They were assured that this administrative implication would be discussed with the proprietors of their health facilities during their own separate training.

Stage 3 update was familiar grounds for the health workers. However, there was additional information that they needed in preparedness for processing those who tested HIV positive through the UCH PEPFAR clinic. The Ogbomoso health facilities had earlier used the Saki referral clinic for their clients. But with changes in the capacity building at various clinics, including in Ogbomoso, it was important that the information they passed on to clients be optimal.

In preparation for their discussion of empowerment for protection from HIV infection, it was clear that the starting positions of the counsellors varied according to their level of education and their pre-update knowledge level about the HIV/AIDS epidemic. Consequently, the approach and methods adopted for the health workers were very close to those of the market peer educators. An additional emphasis was put on work place protection although they were not directly in the caring division of their facilities. Joint MIS training for Peer educators and HIV counsellors

Peer educators that emerged from the review meetings went through 1-day training on record keeping and referrals. The training that was separate for each market, had in attendance ten peer educators and HIV counsellors from health facilities that were attached to the market.

The MIS training was facilitated by the Principal Investigator supported by a Communications specialist who took them through the act of communication. At the end of training a ruled exercise book was given to each of the participants for recording their activities. The IEC department distributed IEC materials to them.

5. The mobilization of materials and resources

A major feature of the APIN project management was the strong emphasis on the biomedical and laboratory aspects of HIV/AIDS control and management. Consequently, the funding of the Virology Department at the UCH meant that laboratory equipment, test kits, and consumables were available for the project. In addition, facilities such as counselling rooms and waiting space were available in each market in preparation for on-the-spot testing and notification of results to volunteers

.

6. The VCT and notification sessions – procedures and management issues

A number of activities on the VCT programme required specialised supervision. The processing of the volunteers and the pre- and post-test counselling were essentially sociological element of the intervention which required limited biomedical information. In contrast, the actual bleeding and testing of samples were based on laboratory and allied disciplines. For this element, the team from the Virology Department, College of Medicine, University College Hospital worked together to facilitate the maintenance of the best practices in the temporary conditions of the market locations. The provision of a well lit and clean room in a house within the market allowed this objective. The oversight of the two sets of activities so that ethical and logistical problems are promptly addressed constituted the third element of the management of the on-site intervention. The resulting efficiencies helped to reinforce the faith of the client in the system. They were assured of the privacy of the counselling situation as well as the confidentiality of the notification of results.

The outcome of this attention to management issues was that at the end of the project, there were no adverse events during the two years. And more impressive still was that given the Yoruba tendency to react in a dramatic and vociferous fashion to adverse news, none of those who tested positive in four markets in Ibadan and Ogbomoso revealed their status to others after the post-test counselling through vocal or body language. This was clear evidence that the aims and methods of the intervention were clearly understood and that the maintaining of test result confidentiality was important to the volunteers. It must be added that some were later involved in sharing the result with others of their own volition when it was advisable to do so for care and support issues arising from the referral system.

Those testing positive in all the markets were referred to the UCH because the conditions in the hospitals in Ogbomoso had not fully met the standards of care and treatment which was then available at the UCH. The fact that members of the HIV testing team were also from the UCH provided continuity of contact in the referral system as ARV clients moved from the market to the PEPFAR clinic at the UCH. One problem that arose from the referral system which was to reduce the regularity of drug pick up as well as adherence to medication was the cost of travel from Ogbomoso to the UCH.

Market based project management – Open market forum

The smooth operations in the market VCT programme were the outcome of the careful attention to details and proactive problem solving approach. Four features of the HIV surveillance, namely, the gathering for public discussion, the processing of volunteers for the VCT, the management of notification of results and the careful attention to ethical issues, were given careful thought and based on previous experience in the management of previous interventions in market places in the earlier phases of the project.

If the project was to generate acceptance among the whole market, the purpose of the bleeding and testing had to be understood by the general market traders. Otherwise, the atmosphere of separateness which could encourage stigmatization of volunteers had to be avoided. Consequently, as in earlier phases, monthly open meetings were following the first general meeting at which approval for the project baseline survey and explanation of the project structure occurred. Subsequently, monthly open market forum allowed the briefing of the market about progress and the fielding of questions as well as the staging of behaviour change without the VCT element for those who attended the meetings. Paying attention to the normal rhythm of the traders allowed the optimization of the meeting times and encouraged people to attend without pressure of trading activities. To make this possible the project team would arrive a day before the meeting and be positioned in the market very early in the morning before farm products arrived in the market. This meant that attendance and participation was always assured. A few items of entertainment obviously helped in making the occasions social whilst being instructive. Provision of chairs and canopies to avoid disruption of procedures when it rained was also attended to.

VCT conducted notification of results, referral and treatment

The first round of VCT was approached with trepidation by the collaborating partners. It was to be a new experience for both partners. For the biomedical teams, some changes had to be made to fit into the arrangements made for confidentiality and informed consent. The hiring of a building in which five rooms and an open corridor were provided for the exercise presented a clinic-type setting rather than an out of clinic exercise. This was good since the corridor served as a waiting space and registration bay. Four of the rooms served as counselling rooms, and one of the rooms served as the bleeding room.

Because of the polyvalence of some of the project staff, it was possible to reduce waiting time for counselling or for bleeding by using some personnel at either task as the occasion demanded. This device was necessary to accommodate the natural impatience that may arise as the traders stay away from their stalls to attend the VCT session. In addition, the arrangement allowed the VCT to take advantage of those periods when the market cycle has not peaked and traders were available for bleeding. The result was an average of 30 to 45 minutes for each client from registration for pre-test, counselling, bleeding and the taking of blood pressure when it is requested by the volunteer.

The initial fear of how readily the first volunteers will turn up was soon allayed. Once the VCT team was in place (very early in the morning by 8.00am) and the project staff had gone around the market with a hailer to inform the market about our readiness, the response was a sight to behold. The market leaders (baba loja, executive members, and some of the trade association leaders) were the first to show up. They assured the team that the others will come in as soon as they arrive in the market. We used the occasion to repeat the message that participation was individual choice with no coercion or loss of privileges. In response the project staff received assurance that there was an eagerness to participate based on awareness of potential benefits rather than pressure being put on anyone. It is worth noting that having the leaders coming in first was consistent with the Yoruba cultural practices of yielding to the elders and leaders the right of first access. That it signals their approval of the process is a supplementary issue that is helpful but by no means coercive.

When within an hour of opening at the very first market, the corridor had more than 10 persons waiting for registration, concern was to make sure that the process will work smoothly. And it did. By the end of 3 hours, 25 people had been bled. At the end of the 9-hour first day the figure of 100 was reached at Aaradaa market in Ogbomoso. The atmosphere was totally relaxed with no sense of anxiety about the process they were to undertake on their faces. Some, however, showed their first reaction to the prospect of being bled when they saw others coming out of the bleeding rooms. It is no exaggeration to state that the atmosphere was relaxed and that people went through the process with their sense of humour and social graces intact. The entire process was not in any way intimidating. That is, in spite of the visible paraphernalia of biomedical project staff in their white overalls, screens to provide functional space partition in the corridor and the formality of going through registration.

Another indication of the state of mind of the volunteers and their preparedness through the training and formative research activities is that only one person refused being bled after pre-test counselling. This refusal was later reversed when the volunteer asked if she could go into counselling again for further clarification. She was granted the request and passed on to another counsellor who was available. She then accepted to be bled.

VCT Procedures

Needless to say, the arrangements for the VCT itself required ingenuity in making the most of the scarce resources in the market for counselling and laboratory work without compromising ethical standards. The innovations included using the project mini-bus as a temporary counselling 'room' in order to reduce the waiting time because of the limited number of rooms available right in the few houses located in the market.

The laboratory staff also utilized the available resources to maximise the efficiency of their operations and necessary resources that could be brought in from the Department of Virology to facilitate their work were made available to them.

The management of notification of results was a potential flash point but in order to minimize compromising the process, additional rooms were provided in a building near the market where the notification could be done with assurance of privacy and confidentiality of the process. In Ogbomoso the set of rooms were adopted for the second, third and fourth rounds of the VCT.

Another strategy employed for the protection of the integrity of project documents was the close supervision of all documentation processes on both the social and biomedical activities. Supervisors had protocols in place for access to project documents and registers so that no unauthorized persons gained access to information which they should not have. Shared confidentiality among the project team itself was kept to a minimum. These precautions did not go unnoticed among the volunteers as they drew attention to some of these during the special review meetings reserved for volunteers only.

There were occasions, though, when the best notifications arrangements get compromised at a later stage. This happens when the volunteers make arrangement for the referral procedures which will mean, for those in Ogbomoso, a day's travel to Ibadan PEPFAR clinic for the follow-up activities arising from their testing positive during the HIV surveillance. Other traders soon notice their absences and make the link with their HIV status. Others also have information about their status revealed by other traders when they meet at the PEPFAR clinic.

The project team's reaction was to stress the issue of sharing of status as a useful strategy for sharing some of the burdens of HIV treatment and management.

Encouraging them to join an emerging HIV support group was part of this strategy. It was out of this initiative that grew the arrangement for group transport as a way of reducing the individual cost of travel to Ibadan. The resolution of the social irritation about positive status was an important element in the credibility of the HIV surveillance process among the volunteers. It made those who tested negative in earlier rounds to continue to repeat the test. The outreach carried out by the volunteer peer educators in the rural markets with which they trade was instrumental in raising the awareness of HIV prevention in general and in spreading the information about prevention and the importance of testing and receiving treatment early in the infection.

7. **The conduct of ten monthly sessions of BCC interventions in open forums in both experimental and control markets so the behaviour modification and change benefits of the project is not denied to the control markets.**

Behavioural change communication in intervention market

Apart from the individual programmes and activities relating to the HIV surveillance, a major component of the project was the creation of the staged behaviour change of the type that was successfully implemented in the earlier phases. For this purpose, an integrated programme of BCC based on the tested methods and materials was implemented in both project towns. However, it was in the control markets only that the series of communication sessions took place. It was the final experimental format for validating the earlier findings on the effectiveness of the 4-stage framework.

The format adopted was the 8 to 10 monthly 2-hour sessions with the wider market audience to which, on ethical grounds, the BCC was targeted. Even if they did not volunteer for the HIV surveillance VCT exercise, they were given the opportunity of being part of the broader objective of encouraging behaviour change and its sustenance in their lives. In addition, the programme created an atmosphere for the development of new norms of behaviour among the traders.

The BCC programme on the project is limited to two intervention markets, one in Ogbomoso and one in Ibadan. That of Ogbomoso market (Aaradaa) took place in the course of the trip. The BCC was based on the four-stage trans-theoretical model, which are

    I.   Awareness creation of the HIV/AIDS epidemic
    II.   Personal risk assessment
    III.   Acquisition of knowledge of risk reduction and avoidance
    IV.   Individual and group empowerment for effective behaviour change

On the basis of previous experience, two sessions each were allocated to the first three stages of the 4-stage framework, namely, awareness creation, self risk assessment and information for effective behaviour change. The last three sessions were allocated to the empowerment needed for implementing necessary behavioural, attitudinal and practices consistent with HIV prevention and proper management.

The first BCC session succeeded in bringing the basic issues of HIV/AIDS prevention as well as the need to make changes in personal behaviour and in the norms and values of societies regarding sexuality to the attention of the variety of sellers. Occasional patrons that passed through the market also listen in on the session and benefited. The second BCC programme was a continuation on the awareness creation of the AIDS epidemic. The forum was also used to mobilize the market for the training of the volunteers who subsequently took part in the VCT exercises. The outcome of the two sessions was the greater awareness and understanding of the epidemic. This understanding generated greater enthusiasm to be part of the project both as volunteers who trained as PEs and those who volunteered to be part of the VCT exercises.

The third of the BCC session was used to emphasize to the audience that everyone is at risk of infection. This activity was used also to demonstrate the relevance of the VCT exercise. Various modes of transmission were discussed with emphasis on the extent to which people may knowingly or unknowingly be at risk. The consensus that emerged from the session was that no one can truly be sure that they are not at risk. These awareness sessions increased interest in the VCT exercises.

The fourth BCC session addressed additional issues raised about vulnerability of individuals. However the session focused the body of information needed to consolidate the third stage of the 4-stage framework. This stage is the acquisition of knowledge of risk reduction and avoidance. Every vulnerability aspect identified in earlier session was reviewed and participants made spontaneous suggestions as to how the risk can be reduced or eliminated. Additional information was provided to supplement their understanding of the issues. The resources that were available to people to effect risk reduction were provided to participants. Those resources included prophylactic methods such as male and female condoms which eliminate the crucial exchange of body fluids during sexual intercourse. Information was provided on where the participants could gain access to condoms and where free supply could be obtained. Information was also made available about health facilities at which STIs could be tested and treated. In addition, participants were informed about the location of HIV VCT services in Ogbomoso and Ibadan.

8   The review of progress made by subgroups of the project participants

From the structure of the project a number of direct and indirect beneficiaries could be identified. These include HIV counsellors from private health facilities, the general market population, the trained market PE volunteers, and all those who took part in the multi-round HIV tests and notification of results. Because of the differences in the composition, roles and knowledge base of the different groups, the progress they made on the performance of the roles and the extent of changes in behaviour were reviewed in separate monthly meetings for the respective groups.

Initially the review meetings were restricted to the volunteers who trained. But after the first round of bleeding, testing and notification sessions, all those who were bled were integrated into these review meetings.

Review session for all that bled

Review meetings of volunteers in each market were put in place to form the basis of sharing experiences among volunteers. The platform was used to encourage the mutual support of the volunteers in adhering to positive behaviour regarding HIV prevention. Synchronising these meetings with the exercise for notification of HIV test results increased compliance with projects' targets and reduced the attrition rate among the volunteers.

Each review meeting was used to assess the retention of training contents and to give updates on the project. As in past reviews, volunteers were given questionnaires to complete. The questionnaire dwelt on the following:
- Rules of disclosure of results
- Appreciation of epidemiology of HIV/AIDS
- Clarifications to learning regarding VCT
- Repeat testing
- Care and support for known HIV positive
- Advanced self risk assessment
- Peer counselling and IEC

As a concession to the varying levels of education of the PEs, the review exercise took the form of a key informant interview with the volunteers making contributions to the questions asked by the PI. The questions asked are broken down into the following:
- The distinction between HIV and AIDS
- The symptoms, care, nutrition and other care of PLWHA
- Condom Negotiations
- Peer Education
- Suggestion for improving the VCT programme

After the review meeting the PEs were given handbills and other IEC materials for their activities.

One-month MIS review with peer educators

The selection of PE and commencement of their activities had to wait till all the IEC materials were prepared. Hence training on the act of communication and record keeping was conducted for twenty volunteers that emerged from a democratic process from the two markets.

As a way of supervising and supporting PEs, a monthly review meeting was put in place. The meeting was to allow the PEs meet to discuss project updates and field experiences, collate the MIS records, solve problems, brainstorm on new strategies and restock IEC materials. The monthly meeting in the future will also be used for specific training in new areas of peer counselling.

The MIS review meetings were held separately at the two project markets. A self-administered questionnaire evaluating what activities they had carried out in reducing the risk of HIV and assessing their own HIV risk exposure was completed by each of the PE's. An interactive session followed the completion of the questionnaire to be able to allow the PE's describe their experience and challenges faced in trying to educate their peers.

Most of the PE's were involved in group discussions rather than in one on one dialogue. These group discussions were carried out in their various religious centres and social gatherings. The one to one education were done with close relations, friends and neighbours they find to be at risk with the exception of one that doubles as a commercial cyclist that uses the opportunity to talk with his commuters which are mostly Ladoke Akintola University undergraduates.

Eight out of the nine PE's trained in Aaradaa market were present at the review meeting. One had relocated to another market. In Ojatuntun all of the PE's were present.

At the end of the meeting, caps and aprons were given to each of the peer educators and their IEC materials were restocked.

HIV Counsellors one month MIS review

Eight HIV counsellors from private health facilities were recruited and trained in pre and post HIV/AIDS counselling. They carried out group and individual counselling within the clinical setup and they were available to the volunteers for any enquiries they had about aspects of the VCT programme and took in referrals generated by peer educators. All eight HIV counsellors were in attendance for the MIS review meeting, as with the Peer educators a self-administered questionnaire evaluating activities they had carried out in reducing the risk of HIV and assessing their own HIV risk exposure was completed by each of them. From the record there were more group counselling sessions than one on one session and these were carried out in religious gathering rather than in the clinical setting.

 The HIV counsellors identified the following as part of the challenges faced in the course of executing their tasks:
- The nurses in doctor owned facilities had little or no contact with the patients.
- Most of the patients were not interested in knowing their status.
- Most referrals generated from the market based PE's could not afford cost for testing and treatment in the private health sector.
- Such referrals are redirected to ARFH in Ibadan and to monthly market activities in Ogbomoso.

In token appreciation of attendance at the review meetings, project caps and aprons were given to each of the counsellors and complementary items were given to the Medical directors/Proprietors of participating facilities.

Use of quiz format in the subsequent reviews

The review of progress among the PE/Counsellors took various forms. The record keeping was reviewed and patterns of errors corrected so as to maintain the quality of the data. But with reference to their knowledge base and retention of learning, a quiz format was devised so as to introduce a competitive edge to the review. Three themes were introduced in the quiz: the HIV risk reduction/prevention among those they counselled, their personal HIV risk reduction in the interval, and their own assessment of what they have achieved as PEs/Counsellors.

During the risk reduction session the respondents were asked if they had counselled anyone on various prevention strategies, namely, abstinence, partner reduction, and condom use. They were also asked if they had referred anyone to clinics for STI treatment or for HIV test and if they agreed to test.

Such was the level of familiarity with open discussion of HIV prevention topics that the PEs/Counsellors thought it appropriate to discuss their own risk exposure. They were, therefore asked to indicate (in writing for confidentiality) if they had been sexually active in the interval and how many sexual partners they had had. They were asked if they had received any injection, blood transfusion or scarification since the last meeting. They were also asked if those who were sexually active used condom only sometimes or not at all.

On some occasions, the review with all those who were bled took account of the mixed educational background by adopting the panel format to the quiz. The facilitator varied the composition by sex and by marital status and each group was given a set of questions which they discussed and had their consensus presented by a member of the group. Each of the questions was to be answered as a group and not as an individual, i.e. they were expected to provide cumulative group answer. This arrangement reduced the personal reservations but provided some amusement when the others try to work out the implications of the answers. For example, a male group made up of two married and one unmarried, and a female group with one married and two unmarried were given the following three questions:

1. How many times have you been sexually active this year?
2. How many sexual partners have you had in the year?
3. Was condom used during the last sexual encounter?

In response the groups gave the following answers:

The male group admitted to have had sex a cumulative total of 8 times in the year 2004 while the female group said their cumulative total was "uncountable". The male group said they had six sexual partners cumulatively within the year 2004 while the female group had three sexual partners. Both groups said they all used a condom the last time. There were instances when the discussion of the responses from the panellists generated additional insight into patterns of behaviour. On another occasion, the male group responded that they had sex ten times in the year while the female group reported 36 times in total. Both sex said they had three partners each. And both groups said they all used a condom the last time they had sex. However, the response of the male was not acceptable to the audience, which prompted the facilitator to ask objections the audience had. In response they were of the opinion that both groups were not saying the truth, because they believe it was impossible for healthy youths to be engaged in sexual intercourse for such low number of times reported by the male whilst the females reported a significantly higher and perhaps more realistic number of times. At the end of the review, IEC materials were distributed depending on the demand from the various PEs and Health Facility Counsellors.

Project team mentoring of HIV positive individuals

A final aspect of the review strategy was the involvement of project team in helping those who tested HIV positive to find solutions to personal or ethical issues arising out of the 6-monthly periodic testing of individuals and the follow up processes involved in referral to PEPFAR clinic in UCH over the 2-year period. In spite of the dignity displayed by volunteers at the time of notification of results, the follow up of referral activities impelled some of those who tested HIV positive to approach members of the project team in confidence on how to resolve some of the problems they faced on account of their positive results.

A number of issues raised in such consultation include the handling of partner notification for those who were married. Another issue frequently raised by volunteers in Ogbomoso was the economic hardship of attending clinic in Ibadan. Others approached team members for the resolution of problems relating to the potential for stigmatization if others in the market knew about their HIV status.

Depending on individual circumstances, the issue of partner notification was usually resolved when the option of couple counselling was offered to those whose partners did not work in the market. Most often the offer was accepted and such partners were offered the opportunity to find out their own HIV status on the project. The economic hardship was resolved when those who attended the PEPFAR clinic realised that quite a number of people from the Ogbomoso markets were HIV positive. From this point onwards it was possible to facilitate the pooling of resources to hire vehicles to take them to the clinic and consequently reduce the cost of travel for clinic appointments. It was the frequent encounter at the PEPFAR clinic that resolved the issue of stigmatization because it became apparent that HIV infection was not uncommon and that those not currently infected had no cause for jubilation as the retention of their negative status required a consistent effort on their parts to stay HIV negative. Also, the level of awareness and behaviour change activities meant that the attitudes in the project markets significantly changed to PLWH.

Adherence to referral appointments and the regular pick up and use of ARV drugs also required the facilitation and reinforcement of instructions by project team members when it was observed from records that some PLWH were not regular in their drug pick-up. This link with the participants also served as a channel of communication between participants and the project sponsors about the challenges they faced and how they believed the sponsors might be able to help.

END OF TRAINING AND END OF YEAR 1 EVALUATION OF PROGRESS ON BEHAVIOUR CHANGE

As a result of the extra vigour put into project implementation on the HIV Surveillance project, it was decided to carry out an evaluation of progress and impact of interventions at the end of the first year. This one year interval also allowed respondents to recall details more accurately than would have been possible at the end of two years.

In an attempt to evaluate the impact of the training session as well as the first year of the market place VCT and the extent to which the volunteers had progressed in behaviour change, a KABP survey of the market was carried out. The sample sizes were set at 666 and 692 in Ibadan and Ogbomoso respectively.

Stigmatization

Significant improvements were registered in the reduction of bias against those who were HIV infected. A decline of 30% and 21% occurred in the proportion of respondents who believed that those who were infected with HIV were necessarily sexually loose. Similarly, there was a decline of 30% and 38% among those who were of the opinion that HIV infected persons were not useful to anyone. Among those who had the judgemental view that HIV infected persons were responsible for own problem, a decline of 17% and 23% was recorded in Ogbomoso and Ibadan respectively. The fatalistic view that HIV/AIDS is a punishment from God witnessed declines of 34% and 21% in the respective towns.

Market place information access

As was to be expected, access to HIV prevention information in the market place more than doubled in the first year of intervention outstripping TV in Ogbomoso. Peer counselling exposure also increased significantly in both towns. The proportion counselled to abstain rose from 55% to 77% in Ogbomoso but with no significant change in proportion in Ibadan where there was an apparent saturation of messages in the market places. In contrast, both towns recorded 15% increase in their counselling encounter encouraging reduction of number of sexual partner. The use of condom also had about the same level of increase in both towns. The most dramatic improvement in HIV prevention counselling in both towns was the advice to test for HIV which rose from 25% at baseline to 77% in Ogbomoso and from 26% to 80% in Ibadan markets.

Measure of progress in translating counsel into action as evidence of behaviour change
When attention was turned to indicators of the ability of the respondents in the target markets to translate knowledge gained into action, the findings were encouraging. The proportion of sample that had ever taken the HIV test rose from 10% to 52% in Ogbomoso and from 12% to 40% in Ibadan. In the context of behaviour change, committing to the HIV test marks a major move towards action that signifies that the staging of behaviour change was about complete in such people.

It was apparent from the baseline information that the amount of knowledge about the epidemic in the markets was such that a felt need for HIV test was existing and that the provision of the opportunity on the intervention was the trigger for action to fill the need. This is the subtle link between stages 2, 3 and 4 of the 4-stage framework. People may feel vulnerable but have no information as to what to do about it. They may also have the information but lack the access to take the test. And, finally, when the test is made available, it requires the courage and inner strength to actually take the test.

Similarly, significant gains were recorded in the use of the male condom by both sexes. At baseline, the proportions of respondents who had used condom with any partner before stood at 17% and 26% in Ogbomoso and Ibadan respectively. But after the first year of intervention, the proportions increased to 43% and 46% in the respective towns. Here again the improvements in Ogbomoso were more dramatic than in Ibadan where message saturation resulted in lower additional gains in behaviour change.

Essence of Stage 4

Two features set behaviour at stage 4 apart from the previous stages. There were measurable indicators to show that action has been taken and for the magnitude of the change. In sexual behaviour, reducing the number of partners, using condom or abstaining, avoiding casual sex, staying within marital sexual activity are examples of such indicators. Table 8.1 below shows the extent of the adoption of the changed sexual behaviour among the sample in both Ogbomoso and Ibadan.

The adopted changes were in specific response to project interventions. In effect, nearly half of respondents had reduced having multiple partners as an HIV prevention strategy. Just under a third had started using condom and a third adopted abstinence. A fifth of the sample avoided casual sex. With the exemption of partner reduction where the proportion making the change was somewhat higher in Ibadan than in Ogbomoso there were no big differences in the responses in both towns to the other indicators of changed behaviour.

Table 8.1: Changed sexual behaviour in response to project interventions

Changed Behaviour	Ibadan	Ogbomoso	Both towns
Fewer partners	41	50	46
Condom use	28	33	31
Abstaining	34	30	32
Avoid casual sex	21	17	19
No extra marital sex	4	0.6	2.4

Source: Survey findings at the end of year 1 (2004).

With regards to non-sexual behaviour changes in Table 8.2, the changes are both interesting and instructive as to how behaviour change information is processed for action. Avoiding the sharing of sharp tools either for pedicure, hair dressing and circumcision was reported by around three-quarters of the sample. Blood transfusion which is less frequently an option is being avoided by about a tenth of the sample. And exposure to non sterile tools in occasional health care contact is also reported by less than 2 percent of the sample. It is apparent that the magnitude of behaviour change is also a function of the extent to which individuals are at risk of the channel of infection.

Table 8.2 Changed non-sexual behaviour

Changed non sexual behaviour	Ibadan	Ogbomoso	Both towns
Avoid sharing sharp tools	72	80	76
Avoid blood transfusion	12	9	10
Test for HIV	5	9	7
Avoid non sterile tools	1	2.4	1.7
Eat good food	1	0.2	0.6

Source: Survey findings at the end of year 1 (2004).

The other vital element of stage 4 is the requirement of effecting behaviour change. That element is the degree of self efficacy possessed by the individual who needed to make the change. This is the evidence to show that the crucial stage 4 had been mastered. The avenue for behaviour change was complete when individuals wished to make such changes. Table 8.3 shows the actions that respondents were able to take or had taken in response to the interventions.

Table 8.3: Changes in self efficacy in response to interventions

	Ibadan	Ogbomoso	Both towns
Discuss HIV/STD prevention with partner	97	86	91
Ask if partner ever had STD	91	81	86
Ask if partner had other sex partner in past 12 months	87	75	81
Convince long term partner to use condom	64	60	62
Convince new partner to use condom	63	55	58
Refuse sex if partner refuses to use condom	58	51	54
Buy male condom in shop	60	53	56
Ask for male condom in the clinic	62	58	60

Source: Survey findings at the end of year 1 (2004).

The greatest gain was in the near universal ability to carry out inter-sexual partner communication about such issues as discussing HIV/STD prevention with sexual partners. Next is the ability to confirm if the sexual partner had any STD history followed by enquiry if partner had other sex partner in the previous 12 months.

Although there is a lower level of efficacy about communications on condom use, yet the levels are significantly higher than what has been reported in national surveys of such communication [NDHS, 2010]. About six in every ten respondents were able to convince long term partners to use condom [64%, 60%], convince new partners to do the same [63%, 55%] and above all refuse to have sex if partner refuses to use condom. With reference to the ability to buy male condom when needed, 60%, 54% were able to do so. About the same proportions were able to ask for male condoms in health clinics [62%, 58%]. These sexual and non sexual behaviour change indices are proof of the validity of the approach to behaviour change which was developed on the series of projects.

ISSUES RAISED BY FINDINGS

A number of observations can be made about the findings to further buttress the evidence for behaviour change. Most volunteers and survey respondents were sexually active adults. Most were linked with others in the sexual network created by the life styles in the market places and the associated activities. Prior to the project intervention, not many considered the taking of the HIV test a priority, either on account of its cost or on account of having no felt need to take one. But through the activities of training, review meetings and voluntary counselling and testing twice in the first year, attitudes changed about the need to take both the STD and HIV tests.

In a significant departure from the shame and secrecy which the test results might attract, people were prepared to share their test results with others, albeit in an orderly fashion moderated by the protocol of the project. Consent of the client was sought before any such notification of others. The sharing was advised to take place in a couple counselling session so that the dynamics of the impact of test result can be moderated by trained counsellors. For most, the project was the first consistent exposure people had about assessing their vulnerability and being encouraged to change behaviour

LESSONS LEARNT ON THE HIV SURVEILLANCE PROJECT

There were five lessons learnt on the HIV Surveillance project. They were:
- That once people are made aware of being at risk and informed about HIV prevention and management services, they are ready to imbibe the habit of regular HIV counselling and testing;
- That the 4-stage framework for BCC programme was instrumental in breaking down the initial scepticism of males, the elderly and the promiscuous;
- That significant sexual risk reduction was documented at project evaluation;
- That above all, once the usefulness of VCT was established in their minds, the volunteers clamoured for the establishment of HCT clinics so that they can continue the habit of regular testing after project cessation;
- That the prompt for the establishment of HIV VCT centres came from the beneficiaries of the project not from ARFH. This was exceptionally rewarding of the effort that was put into the project.

In the next chapter attention is turned to the operations of the HIV VCT centres from July 2005 to August 2013 when competition from improved access to VCT in PHCs and the ending of project support led to the closure of the clinics.

CHAPTER 9
EVALUATING THE IMPACT OF THE 4-STAGE FRAMEWORK THROUGH VCT PATRONAGE

INTRODUCTION

Perhaps the most powerful evidence of the impact of the application of the 4-stage framework in the Ibadan and Ogbomoso APIN sub projects is the level of patronage of the VCT clinics and the evidence of decline in HIV prevalence over the 8 year operations of the two stand alone VCT clinics and at the integrated VCT services provided by the ARFH Main clinic.

Table 9.1 shows the total number of clients tested by year and by clinic site from 2005 to 2014. In total, 39,531 clients patronized the three clinics. Of this number, Yemetu clinic saw 12,001 clients and Ogbomoso clinic saw 9,369 clients. When it is noted that the two clinics operated for only half of 2005 and stopped operations in 2013, and that the ARFH Main clinic records were included only to the middle of 2014, there is evidence that patronage picked up consistently from 2006 to 2009 and declined thereafter when the provision of more HIV testing centres at health facilities in both Ogbomosh and Ibadan meant that fewer clients attended the two clinics.

In contrast, the ARFH Main clinic was complementary to the Yemetu clinic until 2009 when the competition of local VCT services resulted in the decline of patronage at the Yemetu clinic. But with the integration of services at the ARFH Main clinic, patronage picked up and exceeded that of Yemetu every year until the closure of the stand alone clinic. These trends are graphically illustrated in Figure 9.1.

Table 9.1: Total tested by year and by site

YEAR	2005	2006	2007	2008	2009	2010	2011	2012	2013	2014	CLINIC TOTAL
SITE OF CLINIC											
YEMETU	588	1473	1978	2239	1771	1210	1023	1003	716	0	12001
ARFH HOUSE	0	490	633	1238	1615	1603	1667	2624	5639	2657	18166
OGBOMOSO	550	1161	1148	1262	1078	1437	1371	812	550	0	9369
SUM YEAR	1138	3124	3759	4739	4464	4250	4061	4439	6905	2657	39531

Figure 9.1: Total clients tested at three clinics 2005-2013

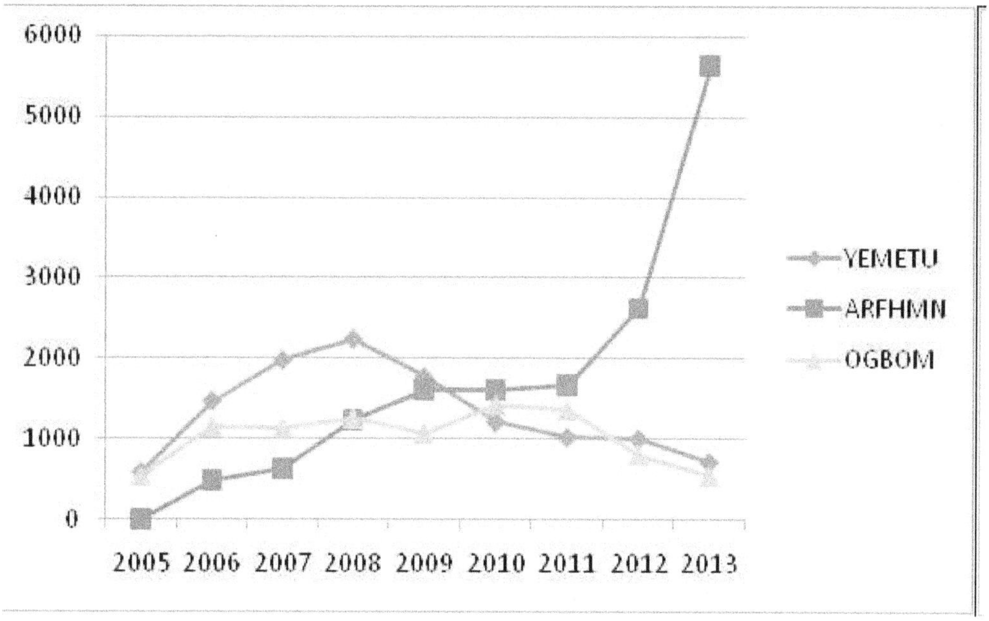

PROPORTION OF REACTIVE TESTS AT THE SITES

Out of the 39,531 tests, a total of 1,659 were reactive. Table 9.2 shows the breakdown of the number by year and site. To appreciate the full import of the data, it is necessary to draw attention to the graphic presentation of the data on Figure 9.2.

Table 9.2: Total reactive by year and by site

YEAR	2005	2006	2007	2008	2009	2010	2011	2012	2013	2014	CLINIC TOTAL
SITE OF CLINIC											
YEMETU	41	67	73	86	64	77	49	37	22	0	516
ARFH MAIN	0	30	28	59	59	64	63	61	84	41	489
OGBOMOSO	87	144	86	92	85	76	45	30	9	0	654
SUM YEAR	128	241	187	237	208	217	157	128	115	41	1659

Figure 9.2: Total clients reactive at three clinics 2005 to 2013

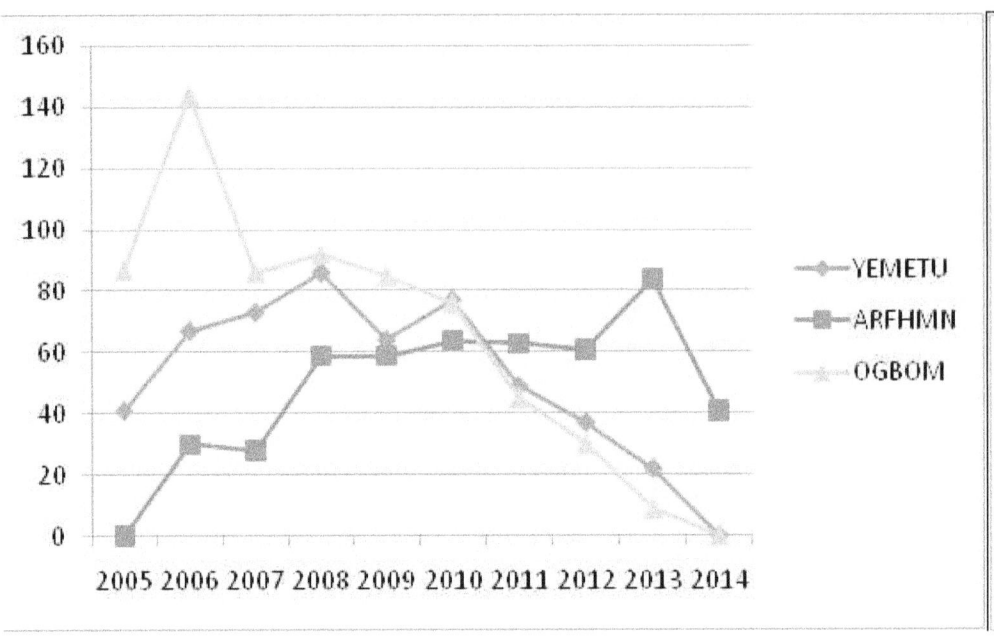

Table 9.3: HIV prevalence by year and by site

YEAR	2005	2006	2007	2008	2009	2010	2011	2012	2013	2014	CLINIC TOTAL
SITE OF CLINIC											
YEMETU	7	4.5	3.7	3.8	3.6	6.4	4.8	3.7	3.1	0	4.3
ARFH MAIN	0	6.1	4.4	4.7	5.8	4	3.8	2.3	1.5	1.5	2.7
OGBOMOSO	15.8	12.4	7.5	7.3	7.9	5.3	3.3	3.7	1.6	0	7
SUM YEAR	11.2	7.7	5	5	4.5	5.1	3.8	2.9	1.7	1.5	4.2

As the prevailing sentinel evidence suggested, HIV prevalence was known to be much higher in the northern area of Oyo State and this was confirmed by the data. The Ogbomoso clinic had a prevalence of 12.4% in the first full year of operations in year 2006 and Yemetu had just over a third at 4.5%. It is noticeable that rates declined systematically in both towns and more so in Ogbomoso than in the Ibadan Yemetu clinic. This produced a convergence of rates at around 3% by year 2012 by which time the prevalence at the Yemetu clinic was the same as at Ogbomoso.

Figure 9.3: Prevalence rates at three clinics 2005 to 2014

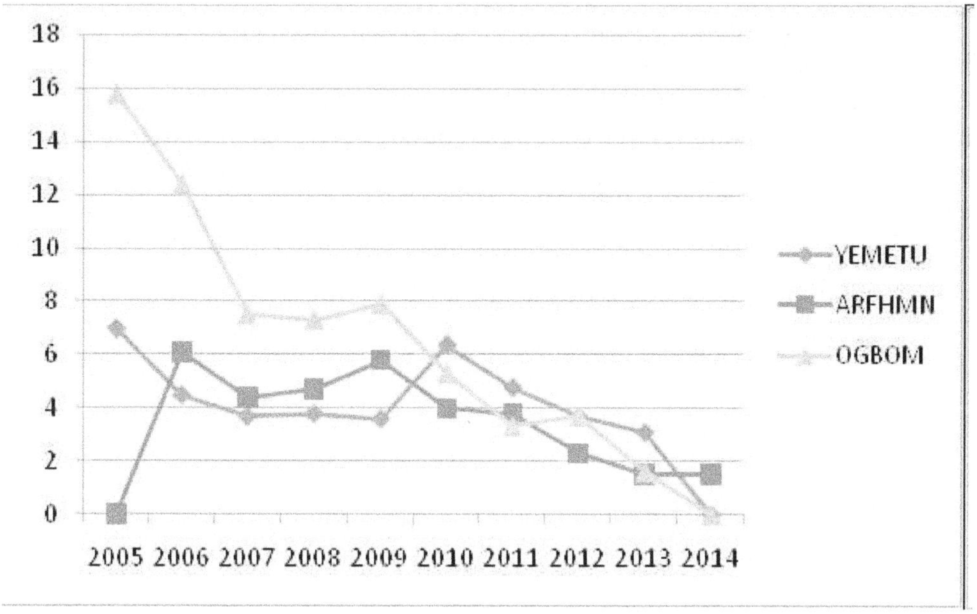

In effect, the outcome of 8 years of consistent testing in both towns reveal that the behaviour change communication in both communities produced a favourable attitude to employing HIV test as a preventive and proactive strategy towards the epidemic. The decline in prevalence from the data cannot be explained by other factors without invoking a real reflection of the changing of the actual prevalence. A case cannot be made that people who know they are positive no longer come to the clinics as there is no way of their knowing unless they test. A suspicion of infection cannot also be given as a consistent explanation for such people to systematically avoid the clinics. To further buttress this line of discussion, results of a sample survey of the sociological factors that may explain the decline are now presented.

INTRODUCTION TO BEHAVIOURAL FACTORS BEHIND TESTING

The ultimate goal of HIV prevention is to alert people about the epidemic, raise their awareness of the personal risks they face and provide them with information on strategies and resources needed to take preventive actions or actions aimed at managing infection. This in effect is the core goal of the 4-stage framework approach. Consequently, when people take the momentous step of taking the HIV test, it is to be interpreted as processing themselves through the four stages of the 4-stage framework. In this chapter, analysis of the clinic records of the three VCT clinics at various phases of the eight years of project operations from 2005 to 2013 allow the logic of behaviour change to be deduced from the information obtained from clinical records and informed consent interviews with a sample of the patients.

The two ARFH implemented APIN project VCT clinics grew out of the HIV Surveillance project in Ogbomoso and Ibadan and were opened in the respective towns on July 8 and July 15, 2005. The period of operation of the clinics fall into two phases which provide different perspectives to the impact of the behaviour change programming that preceded the opening of the clinics. The first four years were operated side by side with continuing activities on HIV prevention projects which reinforced the behaviour change strategies. After 2010, project activities outside the clinic waned with the decline and eventual cessation of funding. By analysing the two segments separately, an attempt is made to show if there is any synergy between project activities and the sustenance of the behaviour change initiatives of clients. In addition, the Executives of ARFH approved the integration of HIV VCT services into the ARFH Main clinic in 2006 and the services are still ongoing beyond the project closure in 2010.

PROFILE OF 3 CLINICS 2005 TO 2009 – SAMPLE OF 2,678 CLIENTS

Sociological survey methodology

In the first four years of the operations of the VCT clinics 15,163 clients were seen in the three clinics. The numbers were 5,199, 5,988 and 3,976 at Ogbomoso, Yemetu and ARFH Main clinics respectively. Of these numbers the sampling procedure for obtaining in depth sociological insights into the profile of clients and the extent to which changed behaviour can be deduced from the profile produced approximately 2,678 interviews in the three clinics. The distribution of the sample was 750, 1,025 and 903 at Ogbomoso, Yemetu and ARFH Main clinics respectively. This produced sampling rates of nearly one in five clients for the three clinics. It was the analysis of this sample survey questionnaire that formed the basis of the additional evidence of the impact of the 4-stage framework on the behaviour change in the clients presented in the rest of the chapter.

Nearly all (95.5%) were new clients. 1.7% were returning for the six monthly repeat tests promoted during the behaviour change processes. the remaining 2.9% gave no response. The highest rate of return was at the ARFH Main clinic with 8% returning for follow up VCT services. This repeating testing was evidence of the attention that people paid to the behaviour change staging.

One other feature of the impact of the 4-stage framework and the attention it paid to both sexes was that the male resistance to sexual and reproductive health issues was reduced. Overall 28.8% of clients were males with 28.5%. 19.1% and 40.2% of Ogbomoso, Yemetu and Main clinics respectively. The 40.2% at the ARFH Main clinic was possibly the outcome of integration of VCT services into the clinic activities which allowed the anonymity of purpose for patronage of the clinic and encourages the attendance of males. The dominance of SRH related patronage of the two other clinics may have discouraged male attendance at the same scale.

A review of the sex composition over the 2008 to 2010 shows that the 2,487 clients, all of whom came to the Main clinic were made up of 25% male at the ratio of three females to one male. The proportion did not radically change in the 2011-2013/14 period when males made up 24.4% of the 46,254 clients at the two Ibadan clinics – Yemetu and Main clinic. In effect, the sex ratio remained constant and could be redressed by finding outlets that blur the SRH image of clinics. This is easier done within the integrated service centres than in stand-alone clinic.

Age composition

Age composition gives an idea of the extent to which VCT services are being accessed by those that have been identified as being at risk, the young and sexually active age groups and others who at a raised risk of infection. Table 9.4 shows that in the 2005-2009 period, the age profile in each of the three clinics was largely similar. Three quarters of clients in each clinic belonged to the 20-39 age group. The proportions ranged from 83.9% at the Yemetu clinic to 70% at the Main clinic.

The under 20s account for around 10% of all clients but their proportion is highest at the ARFH Main clinic at 14.2%. Consistent with the epidemiology of the HIV, persons aged 60 years and above account for less than 2% of the clients.

Table 9.4: Age by VCT clinic

| | VCT CENTRE | | | | | | ALL 3 CLINICS | |
| | Ogbomoso | | Ibadan- Yemetu | | ARFH Main clinic | | | |
	Number	Percent	Number	Percent	Number	Percent	Number	Percent
Under 20	51	6.8	83	8.0	128	14.2	262	9.7
20-29	384	51.2	526	51.3	423	46.8	1333	49.8
30-39	206	27.4	334	32.6	216	23.9	756	28.2
40-49	58	7.7	59	5.7	82	9.1	199	7.4
50-59	25	3.3	14	1.4	40	4.4	79	2.9
60 Plus	23	3.0	9	0.8	9	0.1	41	1.5
No answer	3	0.0	0	0.0	5	0.5	8	0.3
TOTAL	750	100.0	1025	100.0	903	100.0	2678	100.0

Source: Clinical records various years.

Education

The education profile of the clients at the three clinics are shown in Table 9.5 and reveal the strong influence of education level on the assimilation of BCC messages and a positive response to the suggestions made in them. Given the focus on secondary school and post secondary school students in the programmes it is consistent that 88.8% of patrons of the Main clinic have some secondary and post secondary education.

Table 9.5: Education level by VCT clinic

| | VCT CENTERS | | | | | | TOTAL | |
| | Ogbomoso | | Ibadan (Yemetu) | | Ibadan Main clinic | | | |
Education level	Number	%	Number	%	Number	%	Number	%
None	37	4.9	40	3.9	38	4.2	115	4.3
Some Primary	143	19.1	238	23.2	59	6.5	440	16.4
Some Secondary	318	42.4	495	48.3	209	23.1	1022	38.2
Post secondary	237	31.6	250	24.4	591	65.4	1078	40.3
Residual others	12	0.3	0	0.0	0	0.0	2	0.1
No response	13	1.7	2	0.1	6	0.7	21	0.7
Total	750	100.0	1025	100.0	903	100.0	2678	100.0

Occupation

The occupation of individuals is often related to the amount of risk of HIV infection that they carry. The records of HCT patronage reveal that the occupations frequently encountered in the attendance registers were as shown in Table 9.3 for the three clinics during the 2005 to 2009. The Table revealed the dominance of traders, the major group that the APIN/AFRH project addressed. They accounted for 24.8% of the clients. People in paid employment made up one sixth of the clients while students accounted nearly a quarter (23.8%). The high proportion of students is also a reflection of the emphasis placed on the in-school segment of youths during the project implementation. It is also evidence of the effectiveness of the 4-stage framework approach. In effect the three leading groups accounted for nearly two thirds of the clients. The other groups featured included farmers, drivers, tailors and poultry farmers, groups that were also involved in the project activities at the early stages.

Students showed a bias for the ARFH Main clinic and that is to be understood in the context of the Peer Education programmes and 4-stage framework BCC programmes which took place in the premises of ARFH in APIIOS (phase 1 just before the phase II which led to the opening of the HCT programmes). This feature of the patronage lends credence to the thesis that the behaviour change approach adopted on the project was effective in bringing the secondary and tertiary students into the HIV testing habit as a strategy for prevention and management of HIV infection.

Table 9.6: Occupation by VCT clinic

	Ogbomoso	ARFH Main	Ibadan Yemetu	TOTAL
Occupation				
Nothing	3.3%	4.5%	1.4%	3.1%
Trading	37.6%	45.1%	21.0%	34.9%
Tailoring	2.3%	5.9%	1.8%	3.5%
Poultry	3.7%	8.6%	1.9%	5.0%
Farming	3.6%	.7%	2.7%	2.2%
Paid employment	14.3%	12.4%	22.6%	16.4%
Student	15.7%	13.6%	40.0%	23.1%
Apprentice	2.3%	.1%	.0%	.7%
Artisan	4.0%	1.5%	.2%	1.8%
Not applicable	.1%	.5%	.0%	.2%
No response	2.8%	.3%	.6%	1.1%
TOTAL	750	1025	903	2678
TOTAL	100.0%	100.0%	100.0%	100.0%

Client pregnant?

With reference to the link between pregnancy, attendance and pre- and post-natal clinics and the referral of pregnant women to HCT clinics, Table 9.7 shows that around half of the clients of the two stand alone clinics were pregnant women. In contrast, only one in every seven women at the integrated ARFH Main clinic was pregnant. This contrast in part explains why male clients feel more comfortable at the integrated services available at the ARFH Main clinic.

Table 9.7: Client pregnant by VCT clinic

CLIENT PREGNANT?	VCT CLINICS							
	Ogbomoso		Ibadan (Yemetu)		Ibadan (main clinic)		ALL THREE CLINICS	
Yes	322	42.9	594	58.0	123	13.6	1039	38.8
No	419	55.9	429	41.9	780	86.4	1628	60.8
No response	9	1.2	2	0.2	0	0.0	11	0.4
TOTAL	750	100.0	1025	100.0	903	100.0	2678	100.0

TB co-infection

With the established position of TB as a co-infector of HIV, finding out those who had earlier been diagnosed as TB infected was integrated into the processes of HCT. Table 9.8 shows that in the 2005-2009 period about one in twenty clients had been diagnosed with TB before coming to the HCT clinic. The proportion was higher in Ogbomoso at about one in every twelve (8.3%).

Table 9.8: Ever been diagnosed as TB patient by VCT centre

	HCT CLINICS						TOTAL	
Ever been diagnosed as TB patient	Ogbomoso Clinic		Ibadan Yemetu		Ibadan Main Clinic		ALL THREE CLINICS	
Yes	62	8.3	38	3.7	20	2.2	120	4.5
No	668	89.1	983	95.9	882	97.9	2533	94.6
No response	20	2.7	4	0.4	1	0.1	25	0.9
Total	750	100.0	1025	100.0	903	100.0	2678	100.0

HIV Risk Factors

A number of questions were asked from clients to establish the extent of risky behaviour. Table 9.9 reveals that as would be expected from the age profile during this period, over 80% of all clients were sexually active in the previous 12 months. The highest proportion was at the Yemetu clinic at 92.5% and lowest at the Main clinic where just 70% were so sexually active. This pattern again reflects the patronage of the Main clinic where students formed almost half of the clients thus containing a generation that was not as sexually active as the married, pregnant clients in the other stand alone clinics. Consistent with the thesis that the clients had internalized the messages of the 4-stage framework, non response rate was consistently low with just 0.1% not responding to the question.

Table 9.9: Have had sex in the last 12 months by VCT clinic

Sex in previous 12 months	Ogbomoso		Ibadan Yemetu		Ibadan Main clinic		ALL THREE CLINIC	
Yes	618	82.4	948	92.5	629	69.7	2195	82.0
No	130	17.3	77	7.5	273	30.2	480	17.9
No response	2	0.3	0	0.0	1	0.1	3	0.1
Total	750	100.0	1025	100.0	903	100.0	2678	100.0

Number of sex partners

Among the important risk factor in HIV infection is the number of partners. The higher the number, the more likely is the chances of sexual transmission. Those with many sexual partners are by character and circumstances the least likely to regularly use the condom or to use it efficiently. In a series of sex related questions, clients were asked the key risk taking activities they were involved in, and by implication, the need to change to reduce the chances of HIV infection.

Table 9.10 shows that in the 2005 to 2009 period 3.1% of the 2,678 clients stated they had no sexual partner. Just over 60% reported one sexual partner. The highest proportion was 72% for Ogbomoso and an average of 58% for the two Ibadan sites. 11% of Ogbomoso clients reported 2 to 4 sexual partners. The corresponding proportion for Ibadan Yemetu was 30.4%. But in the Main clinic it was 12.2%. Obviously, the clients of the Yemetu clinic appeared to be higher risk takers than those from the other two clinics. The location of the Yemetu clinic near a known sex trade zone may well be a factor in this situation.

Table 9.10: Number of sex partners by VCT clinic

No of sex partners	Ogbomoso		Ibadan Yemetu		Ibadan Main clinic			ALL THREE CLINICS
None	48	6.4	11	1.1	28	3.1	87	3.2
1	541	72.1	600	58.5	516	57.1	1657	61.9
2-3	76	10.1	293	28.6	104	11.5	473	17.6
4+	6	0.8	45	4.5	16	1.9	67	2.4
Not applicable	79	10.5	76	7.4	239	26.5	394	14.7
TOTAL	750	100.0	1025	100.0	903	100.0	2678	100.0

Table 9.11: Number of regular sex partners by VCT clinic

No of sex partners	Ogbomoso		Ibadan Yemetu		Ibadan Main clinic			ALL THREE CLINICS
0	52	6.9	21	2.0	42	4.7	115	4.3
1-2	602	80.3	906	90.4	611	67.7	2119	79.2
3+	14	1.9	16	1.7	5	0.5	36	1.3
Not applicable	75	10.0	69	8.7	236	26.1	380	14.2
No response	7	0.9	12	1.2	9	1.0	27	1.0
TOTAL	750	100.0	1025	100.0	903	100.0	2678	100.0

Heard of condom?

The role of barrier method in the prevention of HIV is well known. The emphasis placed on changing attitude to the product in any behaviour change programme also makes sense. Consequently, it was important to know the extent to which clients have been made familiar with the product and to what extent they have taken on barrier methods as a viable HIV prevention strategy.

Against the background of the emphasis on condoms, knowledge of condom (essentially the male condom) was universal among the clients. In all three clinics,

94.4% reported they had heard of the condom. This proportion essentially covered the clients who were not children.

Unfortunately, knowledge of the condom does not translate into ever using the product. However the proportion of clients reporting ever using the condom was well above what will obtain in the general population. Although most of the clients were in their reproductive ages and in regular unions, some degree of prophylactic use of the condom was being practised. The overall proportion of the 2,678 reporting such use was 46.6%. The site specific proportions were 32.3%, 49% and 55.9% at Ogbomoso, Ibadan-Yemetu and ARFH Main clinics respectively. Here again there was a demonstrable link between education levels of clients and the reported ever use of condom. The frequency of use also varied considerably. Of the 1,259 clients who reported ever using the condom 24% (302) used the condom always. The others used condoms occasionally.

Observations

From the review of the relationships between the profile of clients and the impact of the 4-stage framework, a number of observations are relevant for the first four years of the clinic operations. The behaviour change model certainly made an impact on the male population with a substantial, though not optimal patronage of VCT services by males. The age profile of the clients reflected the epidemiology of HIV. The relationship between education levels and access to behaviour change messages was confirmed by the education composition of the clients over the four years under review. The whole basis of the inadequacy of Western models of behaviour change pointed out in Part 1 is the reliance on the education and knowledge base that members of their public bring to behaviour change communication. The 4-stage framework makes up for that education bias through the staging and the methods adopted for communicating messages in less literate and numerate societies.

Given the attention that was focused on the importance of HIV testing in pregnancy to prevent mother to child transmission of the virus, it is reassuring that the stand alone clinics encouraged the participation of pregnant women in HIV testing at services which were stand alone clinics and served as convenient referral point for the health facilities in both Ogbomoso and Ibadan.

DID BEHAVIOUR AND HABITS CHANGE WHEN PROJECT ACTIVITIES STOPPED?

Although the evidence from clinical records show clearly that the profile of people testing and the outcomes of such tests conform to the known epidemiology of HIV/AIDS in the country, it was largely on the basis of the sociological information collected from a sample of the clients that the impact of the 4-stage framework on the changes made in sexual and other prophylactic behaviour could be argued. It was also mentioned that the period 2005 and 2009 coincided with periods when project activities including the supervision and monitoring of the clinic activities were on going to assure that the standards of operation and ethical issues relating to HIV testing were fully maintained.

In the period from 2010 to end of 2013 the situation changed in terms of the awareness that funding for the operations research attached to the project was ending and that the maintenance of the clinic operations was to continue for a while but come to an end too. Consequently, it came as no surprise that in August 2013, the two stand alone clinics in Ogbomoso and Ibadan closed their doors. As shown in Table 9.1 above the period also witnessed a declining patronage as public sector facilities took on the task of HIV VCT and the processing of those who tested positive into the increasingly robust ARV therapy available in the facilities.

In the discussion that follows, a comparative approach will be used to demonstrate if there are important changes in client's HIV preventive strategies in response to the declining direct programming activities which could be described as confronting the general and special populations at risk of HIV infection.

Volume

During the 2010-2013 period Table 9.12 shows a total of 19,655 clients attended the three clinics and by this period, the ARFH Main accounted for more than half of all clients, a clear evidence that the stand alone clinics were facing a declining patronage because of the increasing opportunities for people to test in other facilities. In order to make the analysis of this post project activity period more rigorous, the sample selection was limited to the two clinics in Ibadan, ARFH Main and the Yemetu clinics. The attendance at the two clinics was 15,465 and from the behaviour survey questionnaire of these a sample of 6,211 was selected at 642/3932 (16.3%) and 5569/11533 (48.2%) in Yemetu and ARFH Main clinics respectively. The higher sampling rate at the ARFH Main clinic allowed a greater confidence in the testing of the hypothesis that with reduction of project activities, the 4-stage framework impact waned.

Table 9.12: Number of clients at the three clinics from 2010 to 2013

YEAR	2010	2011	2012	2013	TOTAL
CLINIC					
YEMETU	1210	1023	1003	716	3932
ARFH MAIN	1603	1667	2624	5639	11533
OGBOMOSO	1437	1371	812	550	4170
SUM YEAR	4250	4061	4439	6905	19655

Age/Sex composition

The selectivity by age continued to reflect the selectivity of the HIV epidemic by age and showed that the under 40 year old dominated the patronage of the clinics. And the cultural factor of male reluctance to associate with sexual and reproductive health issues unless there are pressing personal survival concerns of the time posed by the HIV epidemic maintained a patronage rate of one in every four clients.

Education profile

The education impact on patronage of HIV VCT continues to be important as people with primary school education account for one in eight clients whilst secondary school and university education accounted for 37.8% and 36.8% respectively or for three quarters of all clients.

Table 9.13: Education profile of clients at the three clinics 2010 to 2013

Education	ARFH Main Clinic	Yemetu Clinic	TOTAL
Illiterate	3.3%	2.3%	3.2%
Able to read	.8%	2.5%	1.0%
Primary	11.3%	19.5%	12.2%
Secondary	37.5%	39.6%	37.8%
University/Master/PHD	39.0%	17.8%	36.8%
ND	6.3%	15.4%	7.3%
Total (numbers)	5569	642	6211
Total (percentage)	100.0%	100.0%	100.0%

The major development in this second phase of the clinic services is the increase in the proportion of clients with post secondary/university education. This is consistent with the observation that the clients of the ARFH Main clinic tended to be better educated than those of the community based stand alone clinics.

Occupation

The differences in occupation profile in the second phase of the Ibadan clinics can be seen within the framework of the increasing shift of some occupations to the ARFH Main clinic. Students maintained their proportion of clinic patronage but there was a sharp decline in the patronage of the ARFH Main clinics by the trading/business community. From 45% in the 2005 to 2009 period, there was a decline to 28.8% in the proportion of the traders using the clinics. It is possible to postulate that this is the market based community who may be shifting their patronage to the local health facilities that were offering HIV VCT services from 2010 onwards. In contrast, the level of patronage of the Yemetu clinic by the traders stayed steady at 28.8% and 29.6% for the respective phases of the analysis.

Table 9.14: Occupation of clients at the three clinics 2010 to 2013

Occupation	ARFH Main	Yemetu	Total
Unemployed	2.3%	5.8%	2.7%
Artisan	10.4%	9.8%	10.3%
Business/Trading	28.6%	29.6%	28.7%
Civil Servant	6.3%	7.5%	6.5%
Student	15.2%	19.9%	15.8%
Lecturing/Teaching	8.2%	5.0%	7.8%
Health worker (Doctor, Nurse)	2.4%	1.6%	2.3%
Retired/Pensioner	.4%	.3%	.4%
NR	11.2%	5.1%	10.4%
Total (Count)	4455	642	5097
Total (Percentage)	100.0%	100.0%	100.0%

HIV Risk Factors

Apart from the demographic profile of clients, the real issue of importance to the evaluation of the impact of the 4-stage framework is to find out if the risk factors changed negatively during the second phase. There was no significant difference in the proportion of those who ever had sex. Nor were there significant differences in the number of sex partners reported in the 2010-2013 phase.

With reference to the development of risk reduction plans, a large difference existed between the 56.5% of ARFH Main clinic clients who had developed such plan and the 86.9% of Yemetu clients who had such plans developed. The difference cannot be explained in terms of personal characteristics such as age, sex and marital status. Education should have made the ARFH Main clinic clients more proactive, but that did not happen, suggesting that there are other explanations for this difference. A worrying possibility is that the more sophisticated clientele may be relaxing their guards because they may have confidence in their increased knowledge base and in the degree of control they have on their actions as a result of the internalization of the implementation of the self risk assessment based 4-stage framework approach. Clients at Yemetu are not more involved in at risk activities than other groups at the other clinics.

Observations

With the range of personal characteristics and behaviour that VCT clients presented in this evaluation of the 4-stage framework, there is reason to accept that it is a viable option for staging behaviour change in the circumstance of an epidemic such as the HIV/AIDS. The staging process also appears logical and convincing to the target population. Equally important is that once the services are in place to support the behaviour change goals and objectives, the public will respond positively to the prevention of infection.

The issue of funding the initial process of operations research into this 4-stage framework approach is important to understand. The time required for working out the processes of change is both time and resource intensive. It was fortunate that ARFH found in APIN a sponsor for those sub-projects which collectively allowed the development of the 4-stage framework approach in as varied a social and epidemiological setting which underpin the robustness of the model.

One of the most astounding coincidences of the circumstances of publishing this book is that unavoidable delays resulted in the outbreak of Ebola Virus Disease in the West African region. That outbreak came in such a form as to allow a confrontation of the issues raised in chapter 1 when a distinction was being made between outbreaks of diseases and epidemics. It is therefore, inconceivable that the book should be published without discussing how the similarities and differences between HIV and EVD reinforce or undermine the 4-stage framework approach to behaviour change. In the final chapter therefore the course of the EVD outbreak and how those similarities and differences affect the process and mechanisms as well as the ethics of behaviour change form a post-script to the book.

CHAPTER 10
THE NIGERIAN EBOLA VIRUS DISEASE OUTBREAK

INTRODUCTION

P rior to July 20, 2014 when the index patient arrived in Nigeria, the current West Africa Ebola outbreak, the worst in the history of the EVD was not high on the list of Nigerian public health priorities. The preoccupation was with the ongoing HIV epidemic and the upsurge in insurgency by the Boko Haram. In any case, the characteristic optimism of Nigeria led to the conclusion that bad events somehow pass over the country. Consequently the Nigerian media concern for the West Africa EVD outbreak was limited to the reporting of its extent and intensity in the three countries affected, namely, Guinea, Sierra Leone and Liberia. There was also a limited dissemination of broad outlines of modes of transmission and prevention. On July 20, 2014 when the index case flew into Nigeria, the only mention of Ebola was a short health piece by Fabian Odum on the summary details of the outbreak. He described it as the deadliest in the 38-year history of the epidemic. There were 932 cases and 615 deaths or a fatality rate of 65.7% as of that date (*The Guardian*, July 20, p. 14).

Another public health concern on that date was the ongoing Resident Doctors' strike which was at the time in its third week focusing attention on the general malaise of the Nigerian health sector. Ironically, a day after the arrival of the index patient, Patrick Sawyer (PS), the health issue in the Guardian newspaper was the sorry state of the Nigerian health care system written by Dan Nwomeh and citing the current WHO ranking of Nigeria health care system as 187th out of 190 countries, and only ahead of Democratic Republic of Congo, Central African Republic and Myanmar [*The Guardian*, July 21, pp. 84-85].

In an unusually smooth collaboration between the Lagos Government agencies, especially the MOH and the Federal MOH and partner local and international organisations such as the WHO, CDC, and the Nigerian Centre for Disease Control, within eleven days of arrival of PS, the following dramatic but extremely effective steps had been taken to contain the spread of the virus.

With obvious collaboration between airport health authorities and public health officials, the tracking of primary and secondary contacts of PS was initiated and reported in the press. One feature of the immediate responses to the news of the entry of Ebola virus into Nigeria was the focus on public health institutions and health agencies taking responsibility for the protection of Nigerian citizens from the immediate threats of the EVD. This element of the outbreak touches more on policy and programmes for public health than on the individual responsibility for assuring personal health through behaviour change. The personal responsibility phase followed thereafter. The public awareness information was the orderly aspect of the personal health responsibility. But the disorderly personal response was driven by the fear induced by the parameters of the new virus. It reminded one of the early days of HIV when initial focus was on the ultimate fatality of the infection because progression took so long and was ever so variable a time period from individual to individual. Over the years the perception of the HIV changed as improvements in antiretroviral drugs changed the "death sentence" image of HIV.

Pace of the West African outbreak

The next phase of the Nigerian Ebola outbreak was the unfolding in the newspapers of the impact of a single index on the psyche of the nation. A day before the death of PS the only Ebola piece in the Guardian newspaper was on the EVD infection of Sierra Leone's Chief Ebola doctor. Quoting the report from WHO of July 19, 2014 the piece put the current fatality rate at 60% much lower than the high end estimate of 90% in some earlier EVD outbreaks. The pace of the epidemic revealed in the WHO report indicated 19 new deaths and 67 new cases were recorded within the four days since its previous statement. The pace of new infections and deaths was to pick up considerably in the months of August and September with an estimate of 40% of all known cases in the three worst affected countries coming up within 6 to 8 weeks following the arrival of Ebola virus in Nigeria. As will be discussed later, the confluence of the Nigeria outbreak and the turn for the worse of the West African outbreak raised the profile of the EVD outbreak as well as the urgency of the responses from various countries and regions of the world.

With the increased coverage of the Nigeria outbreak, the dailies started devoting space to some exotic features of the origin of the Ebola virus. The Natural Health section of the Guardian newspaper did a full exposé on eating bush meat as "viral feast". Mention was made of bitter kola, garlic and other products touted as offering protection against the Ebola virus (*The Guardian*, July 24, 2014, pp.9, 43-44 and 46).

On the same date, the Senior Special Assistant to the Lagos State Governor on Public Health, Dr. Yetunde Adesina, gave a press briefing in which she referred to the start of the West African outbreak in March 2014 in Guinea, Liberia and Sierra Leone. It turned out that on July 22, 2014, the third day of PS arrival in the country, the First Consultants Medical Centre (FCMC) contacted the Lagos State MOH when EVD was suspected. She referred to PS's claim of no previous EVD contact in Liberia. But because of his residence in an endemic region and "presentation of non-specific constitutional symptoms and signs of fever, malaise, body aches, vomiting, diarrhoea, etc associated with EVD, a high index of suspicion was raised." Consequently, the patient was admitted and detained and blood samples sent to the Virology Reference Laboratory, LUTH, and WHO Reference Laboratory in Dakar, Senegal. As a result of palliative care initiated by FCMC the patient was stable, vomiting stopped; intravenous infusion had also been stopped and Universal Safety Precautionary Measures to prevent spread of disease and guarantee the safety of other patients put in place in the hospital [*Nigerian Tribune*, July 24, 2014, p.9].

At this stage, public attention was focused on the symptoms and presumed "cure" or "treatment" for Ebola virus. This marked the first stage of people taking personal responsibility for preventing infection. But because of some miscommunication, some comical and dangerous changes in behaviour were embarked upon with equally serious consequences on the health of individuals.

Some changes in behaviour based on misinformation

The early weeks saw the mass media dissemination of the basic elements of the sources of the Ebola virus, the human to human pathways of transmission and significant confusion as to how it can be managed or "cured". The print media in particular depended on three sources of information. The WHO regular EVD updates focused on the numbers of identified cases and known deaths at specific dates especially for the core EVD countries. Others use some sociological insights as to how the outbreak is fuelled by such cultural practices as intimate caring of the sick, elaborate funeral rites and the unfamiliar and alien concept behind the process of quarantine and refusal of contacts to the suspect patients or those infected with the Ebola virus. To these sources must be added the informed or uninformed views of commentators in the media:

> Exposure to infected people as families care for sick relative at home, touching bodies during burials or even nosocomial (hospital-acquired) infections continue to account for the high death tolls. One WHO estimate suggested that as much as 60% of transmission in the three countries were the result of such contacts with infected individuals or with dead patients when they are particularly contagious. However, according to the Food and Agric Organisation rural communities still hunting for bush meat risk further spill over of the virus from infected wild animals [*Nigerian Tribune*, August 9, 2014, p. 6, 5, 1].

> In effect, the EVD, like HIV/AIDS, touches on the deep seated habits of people within their communities and makes more difficult attempts at changing of behaviour. The social activities that make life meaningful are the very ones that epidemics and outbreaks undermine. In spite of the serious concerns expressed by the Lagos State Government about the potential risks of large gatherings and excessive physicality of social interactions, Lagos State residents ignored the warnings and continued to meet in crowded places. Food is displayed in unhygienic conditions in markets and handling of products by potential buyers continues without consideration for the exposure of individuals to body fluids of others in the process [*Nigerian*

Tribune, August 9, 2014, p. 7].

> Although the HIV was initially perceived as a contagion which prompted the phase of stigmatization and physical avoidance, the backlash to the American/Liberian carrier of EVD into Nigeria was the emergency of stigmatization of Liberians, prompting the ambassador of that country to appeal for understanding *[Nigerian Tribune, August 9, 2014, p. 9].*

Far worse was the discrimination of categories of people presented in media reports as particularly vulnerable. These categories include health workers and commercial motor cyclists (popularly known as "okada").

In Kogi State some landlords were alleged to have ejected health workers and commercial motor cyclists shun them to avoid intimate contacts of the type that general information warned against. The State MOH tried to allay the fear of outbreak in the state [*The Guardian,* August 20, 2014, p. 7]. Other forms of stigmatization came from unexpected quarters. Panic reaction to people who showed signs of fever emerged because of inadequate knowledge of the Ebola virus. Medical personnel were reported to be running away from patients with such signs instead of taking care of them as appropriate [*The Guardian*, August 20, 2014, p. 18].

The same panic led to rapid adoption of salt/salt bath as cure/prevention. The desperation behind the panic was expressed in these terms on the opinion pages of a newspaper:

> "I think the citizenry has enough reason to panic even now. In a country where health care delivery system is very poor, where doctors are on strike for months on end and the sick are left to die, where drugs, medical supplies and other medicaments and facilities are in short supply and not affordable where they exist, the thought of a ravaging disease with no sure cure is debilitating and shocking." [*Nigerian Tribune,* August 20, 2014 p. 20 - Opinion page piece by Nasamu Jacobson]

First Consultants Medical Centre Ltd, Ikoyi Road, Obalende, Lagos, gave the time of death of PS as 6.50am on July 25, 2014. Dr Adadevoh, the Lead Consultant who was in charge of his treatment mentioned the role that refusing the extraction of PS by his diplomatic handlers so that he could travel to Calabar played in curtailing the spread of the virus.

Additional evidence of the deception on part of PS emerged. He was reported to have denied contact with Ebola patients in Liberia when in fact his sister had died earlier of the disease. When he did not respond to malaria treatment and tested negative for HIV and hepatitis B and C, his samples were sent out for test for the Ebola virus. Result from LUTH signalled PS infected with Ebola virus – Zaire strain. Confirmation of result was conducted in Senegal WHO Reference Laboratory, at the Redeemer's University in Ogun State and at LUTH, Lagos. This networking with international agencies and alerting other countries (Togo stopover) was a hall mark of the Nigerian response.

In the meantime, evidence of the extent of PS deception emerged elsewhere: Sawyer knew he had contracted Ebola before coming to Nigeria: In an article published on its website, a Liberian newspaper, The New Dawn, reported that CCTV footage from the James Sprigs Payne Airport in Monrovia showed that Patrick Sawyer was visibly ill before his flight. The footage reportedly showed Sawyer avoiding bodily contact with other travellers and airport officials. "His face bore a sad countenance like someone who was troubled," the article wrote. It added that the video showed Sawyer "lying flat on his stomach on the floor in the corridor of the airport, a sign of someone in excruciating pain." People reacting to the report, expressed anger that the Liberian did not take adequate measures in consideration of others' health, especially as his sister had succumbed to the disease [*Nigerian Tribune,* August 8, 2014. p. 4].

The airline industry response included the screening of all inbound passengers. Airline that makes 80 or more trips to Nigeria were also alleged to have been suspended. ASky Airline that flew in PS from his transit stop in Togo was suspended and asked for evidence of capacity to prevent recurrence if it was to continue flying into the country (*Nigerian Tribune,* July 29, 2014, pp. 2, 4).

What the Nigerian outbreak did for the international profile of the West Africa outbreak was to draw a dramatic attention to the potential for the outbreak to become an epidemic. A single infected person arrived in the country caused such a furore that people started paying attention to details of the larger West African outbreak.

One of such details of the larger outbreak was the report of the US doctor who contracted the EVD in Liberia and had to be repatriated to the US for treatment using a trial drug that had not been approved for use in humans. The other was the report that a Sierra Leone woman who fled hospital after diagnosis died in Freetown, becoming the first confirmed case in the Sierra Leone capital where there were no facilities to treat the patients with EVD.

These episodes drew attention to vital elements of the management of the Ebola virus outbreak as well as the unfolding Nigerian outbreak. First, air travel could be a vehicle for dissemination of the virus to a wider area of the world. Second, the neglect of drug development for the EVD by pharmaceutical companies, just because the numbers of people affected were few and in non-strategic parts of the world was a short sighted policy. Third, the draconic measures of quarantine and other forced behaviour changes required for preventing spread of infections required a new mind set as to what methods and procedures could legitimately be required for behaviour change in such extreme health emergency. And fourth, that global leadership by the WHO was going to be an important element in managing the rapidly transforming outbreaks.

WHO response

The overall impression was that the WHO was slow to recognise the seriousness of the West African outbreak even though the charity Medicine Sans Frontier (MSF) had raised an alarm suggesting that the outbreak was out of control. The WHO declared a global emergency on August 8 [*Nigerian Tribune*, August 9, 2014, p.4]. The World Bank set aside emergency fund towards Ebola response [The Guardian, August 8, 2014, p.31]. The full text of the WHO Global Risk Statement was made available in the press the next day [*Nigerian Tribune*, August 9, 2014, p.48]. As subsequent updates on the outbreak revealed, the World Health Organisation underestimated the severity of the outbreak and some of the criticisms were valid.

United States Response

It is important to mention that the infection of a US doctor in Liberia and the arrival of EVD in Nigeria by air prompted a raised level of priority attached to the EVD by the United States government. The former raised the issue of national interest whilst the Nigerian outbreak demonstrated the potential for dissemination of the outbreak through international travel and in particular by air travel. Subsequent isolated cases of repatriation and arrival of infected individuals in the US and varying degrees of host health facility preparedness to handle the patients created a furore about the handling of the EVD as a global as well as national health emergency in the United States. In fairness to the US, once roused, it played the role of galvanising Western support for the effort to assist the core affected countries to tackle the outbreak. In this role, she found ready support and independent energies in the Government of the United Kingdom. The self interest in tackling the outbreak "at its source" makes sense given the success of the Nigerian effort at controlling the spread of the outbreak beyond the final tally of 20 infections and 8 deaths and the successful treatment and clearing of infection in the 12 survivors.

Local and international perception of the Nigerian response

In spite of the coherence of the management of the outbreak by the Lagos and Federal MOH, it appeared the public was not assured because of the prevailing perceptions of the limitations of the local health services:

> Survey reveals 72% of Nigerians lack confidence in the capacity of local hospital to manage the disease; 91% aware of outbreak; 82% more concerned about EVD than other diseases such as HIV (8%), Hepatitis (3%); 57% have confidence in the FMOH and agencies to manage the outbreak (poll week of Aug 11, 2014 conducted by NOI Polls Ltd) [report by Emeka Anuforo, *The Guardian*, August 20, p.7 and *Nigerian Tribune*, August 20, 2014, p. 41].

In much the same way an Editorial titled "Innovative actions before it is too late" drew attention to the state of the health system, confusion about various experimental drugs and reference to the Italian doctor Bernadino Ramazzini (Nov 3, 1633 to Nov 5, 1714) who discovered quinine from the bark of cinchona as cure for malaria. The editorial advised that Nigeria should seek help from people who have experience dealing with the disease and not waste money on pesticides (sanitizers). The strike of the Nigerian Medical Association was contrasted to Emory staffers in the United States who did not go on leave until the infected American arrive the US. The gratitude due to the staff of the First Consultants Med Centre and to Dr Stella Adadevoh who recognized the Ebola infection in Sawyer and stayed on to manage the patient and eventually died of her intervention was also remarked on [*The Guardian*, August 20, 2014, p. 16].

Federal and State Government Responses

Against the background of the scepticism of the Nigerian public, it is worthwhile doing a brief review of the Federal and State government responses that was to produce the control of the outbreak which resulted in the WHO declaring Nigeria free of Ebola on October 20, 2014. In the first few weeks after the start of the Nigerian outbreak, attention of both the State and Federal medical authorities and agencies as well as the general public turned to the peculiar features of the Ebola virus which set it apart from the HIV virus and implied a new learning curve was required if the new and more present danger of Ebola virus was to be avoided.

In spite of the high mortality attributed to Ebola virus put at between 60% and 90% in the current West African outbreak, the fact remained that not all die within the dramatic 21-day frame used as justification for the length of the quarantine period. According to <livescience.com> "A minority recover from infection difficult to predict who will survive. Infection depletes the body's immune cells in particular CD4 and CD8 T lymphocytes, which are crucial to the functioning of the immune system (Derek Gathere, a bioinformatics researcher at Lancaster University, UK)". In other words, there were some striking similarities between the pathways of destruction of the immune system by both the HIV and the Ebola viruses.

Another ray of hope came from the fact that "Two US workers who contracted Ebola in Liberia improved after receiving an unapproved drug, ZMapp developed by the Mapp Biopharmaceutical based in San Diego, United States." [*The Guardian,* August 8, 2014 pp. 28, 29].

The first policy priority for Nigeria was how to tighten the entry conditions from abroad either by air or land so that the PS escapade is not repeated. It was disheartening that PS, in spite of his level of information about the EVD and his personal impact of the epidemic as well as his own infection, took the unusual though it turns out human reaction to danger by disobeying the most elementary of scientific advice. Other medical personnel directly involved in the containment of the Nigerian outbreak took the same strange behaviour of eluding quarantine to travel to Port Harcourt and other parts of the country. These reactions to danger put a new light on the PS travel to Nigeria. It could be true, as the wife suggested in an interview with NBC TV in the US that he came to Nigeria to access what he believed to be a superior health care system than that of his country Liberia. Although he died soon after arrival, the heath care system has shown itself to be better than the war ravaged health care system left behind after years of civil war in Liberia.

This pattern of behaviour by well trained and informed health workers and other individuals reinforce the energy and persistence required in attempts to change human behaviour in epidemics or outbreaks. It also demonstrates the clash between common good and personal priorities when behaviour change may be good for society but not in the best interest of the individual.

As a direct measure of containment of the virus, the ECOWAS in Lagos was shut down for necessary decontamination. Meetings were suspended and some of their officers were placed under surveillance. Boarder authorities were to start screening outbound passengers; Nigerian Ports Authority placed medical team on alert and rolled out guidelines for the processing of passengers at the points of entry and departure [*The Guardian*, August 8, 2014, pp. 1, 2 and 6].

Medical experts in aviation held sensitisation seminars and warned that panic was more dangerous than the disease – "malaria kills over 1000 people daily yet no attention, but because EVD kills and very few survive the infection it attracts more attention" [*Nigerian Tribune*, August 18, 2014. p. 42].

State governments moved to stop outbreak. UCH was to assist in testing blood samples. The Lagos government urged cancellation of religious crusades. Ogun and Kogi states emphasized that there were no cases in their states. In the meantime the public was cautioned about the emerging half truths and outright myths about the efficacy of salt solution and bitter kola. In response to these unproven "cure", the Federal MOH advised against chewing of bitter kola since the study of the effect was inconclusive [*The Guardian*, August 20, 2014, p. 1]. Anambra State government procured kits for medical personnel to be involved in Isolation centres. Delta State government set up crematoriums to handle the destruction of dead bodies which was claimed to have fuelled the Liberia outbreak when relatives went through burial rites. Kaduna State government warned citizens to be on the alert for signs of the Ebola virus in their interactions. Regional groups of states held joint meetings on how to contain the outbreak. One such meeting was held between Lagos, Ogun and Ondo States.

Other measures included Ogun State government purchasing protective equipment; Ondo State government designating 3 hospitals in different zones of state to handle the quarantine of suspected contacts of people infected with Ebola virus. Committees of doctors, nurses and laboratory personnel were also set up. Nurses were trained on barrier nursing. Kano State also designated hospitals for quarantine and treatment. Delta State set up special wards in hospitals. Kwara state was keen to declare its Ebola free status [*Nigerian Tribune*, August 8, 2014, p.47].

The Federal Government on its part announced insurance for health workers when it was apparent that they faced risks beyond the normal call of duty, and more protective equipment were ordered to meet the rising needs for these disposable outfits used for close care of those under surveillance or treatment [*Nigerian Tribune,* August 8, 2014, pp.1, 4].

Enforcement of Behaviour Change as response to Ebola virus

With the heightened attention on the West Africa outbreak, a number of behaviour control measures were put in place in the worst affected countries. In Sierra Leone security forces imposed complete blockade on the eastern areas hit by Ebola. Movement out of Kenema was restricted and only essential goods were allowed into the town at the intersection of the three countries of Guinea, Sierra Leone and Liberia [Al Jazeera TV]. From September 16 to 19, 2014, Freetown was in lockdown and people stayed indoors so that teams of health workers could visit every home to take temperatures, identify people who are showing symptoms and take them and their contacts into quarantine.

Figure 10.1: 2014 Ebola Outbreak in West Africa - Outbreak Distribution Map

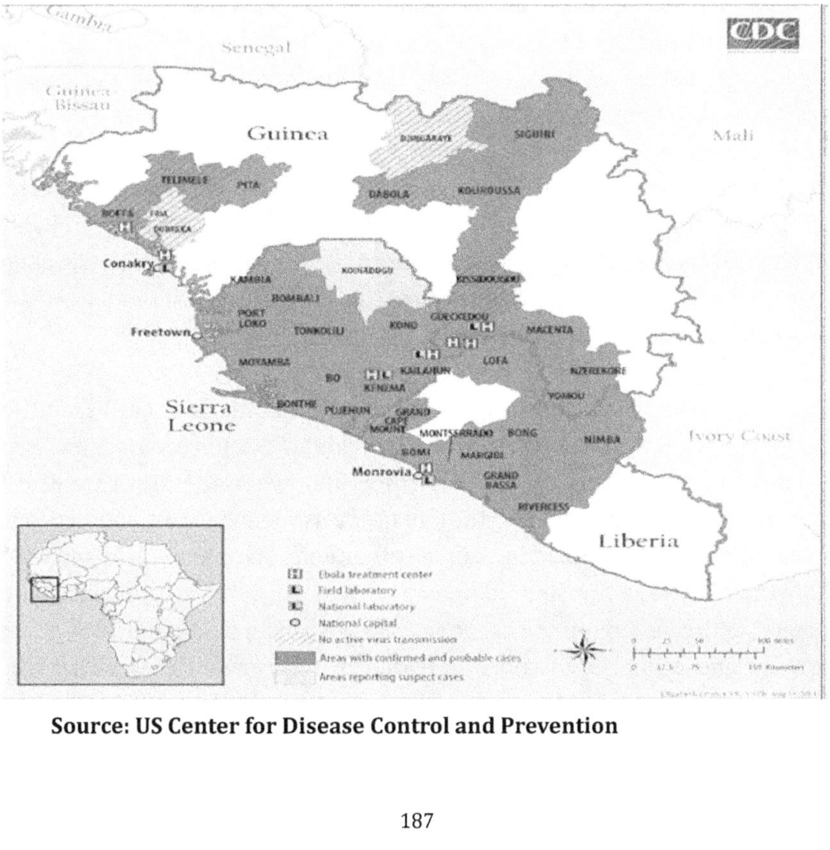

Source: US Center for Disease Control and Prevention

The Liberia government declared a state of emergency in the country [The Guardian, August 8, 2014, p. 6]. Liberian soldiers set up road blocks stopping people from the affected western area of the country from moving into the capital Monrovia [*Nigerian Tribune*, August 8, 2014, p.49].

In fairness, at the end of the Freetown lockdown exercise, 136 individuals with symptoms of EVD were identified and taken into care. In effect, harsh as the lockdown was, it contributed to the control of the spread of the EVD in Freetown. However it does not detract from the harshness of quarantine which denies individuals of a cherished human trait which is to be in the company of relevant others. It is at this point that it should be mentioned that one country employed quarantine as a tool of HIV/AIDS prevention in 1986. The account of that Cuban experiment is worth mentioning in detail:

The Cuban quarantine policy for HIV from 1986 to 1994

As soon as AIDS reached Cuba, the Cuban government, through the Ministry of Public Health, designed and implemented national programme aimed at controlling the spread of disease. Cuba's strategy differed enormously from other nations and was legally founded in already existing regulations to protect citizens' health. Regulations included: Decree-Law 54 of April 1982 stating that, "for the exercise of prevention and control actions for communicable diseases, one or more of the following measures will be adopted, depending on the case: isolation of individuals suspected of suffering from a communicable disease, and of possible carriers of the causal germ, if necessary, as well as the suspension or limitation of these individuals' activities when their realization poses a risk for the health of others."

Furthermore, Law 41, of July, 1983, on Public Health, whose article 20 referred to diseases that might become epidemic stated that, "the Ministry of Public Health will determine which diseases pose a risk for the community, will adopt diagnostic and preventative measures and will establish methods and procedures for mandatory treatment.

These regulations led to the lawful creation of the Santiago de Las Vegas AIDS Sanatorium in Havana for HIV -positive individuals. Similar sanatoriums were created in other areas of Cuba. So from 1986, when the first case of HIV appeared on the island, to 1994, the Cuban government quarantined all people found to be HIV infected. In the sanatoria, patients learn about HIV and AIDS, how the disease is transmitted, how a person can prevent transmission to others, and safe sex practices. Food, housing, medication, social services, privacy, and other services are provided in the sanatoria, as well as the intensive educational and preventative programme (Hoffman, 2004).

Does the end then justify the means? This is an issue to which the concluding remarks at the end of the chapter will return in the context of the relevance of the 4-stage framework to the peculiar features of the EVD. In the meantime, the ethics surrounding the development or non development of drugs and vaccines for EVD until recent events and the potential for the global spread of the disease triggered reactions from the WHO to the World Bank and the United Nations.

The ZMapp trial treatment for EVD

As hinted above, the slow pace of development of drugs for the management of the EVD was a natural geo-political reaction to the profit motive behind most commercial venture in the developed countries. Consequently, knowing that the ZMapp was possibly an effective treatment and knowing that some US citizens infected in the West African outbreak were treated with the drug did not help the sense of disbelief in the affected African countries. The US President justified his refusal to authorise the release of the drug to be sent to West Africa in the following terms:

> It is premature to send Ebola drug to W/Africa: He said he lacked enough information to green-light a promising medicine called ZMapp that was already used on two American aid workers who saw their conditions improve by varying degrees.

> "We got to let the science guide us and I don't think all the information is in on whether this drug is helpful." Obama said. "The Ebola virus, both currently and in the past, is controllable if you have a strong public health infrastructure in place." "But, he said: "the countries affected are the first to admit that what's happened here is the public health systems have been overwhelmed. They weren't able to identify and then isolate cases quickly enough." "As a consequence, it spreads more rapidly than has been typical with the periodic Ebola outbreaks that occurred previously" [*Nigerian Tribune,* August 8, 2014, p.49].

On its part the WHO grappled with the ethical issues of approving ZMapp for human use by stating on August 6, 2014 that it would ask medical ethics experts to explore emergency use of experimental treatments. Although as morally expected the group did approve that the circumstances warranted the use of experimental drugs. However, the hope generated by the decision was dashed when it emerged that the manufacturers of the ZMapp drug, the most prominent of the experimental drugs, stated that the experimental drug was exhausted [*The Punch,* August 13, 2014, front page]. The only ray of hope came from the WHO about the possible fast tracking of drug development which could make some vaccines available for early 2015 [*Nigerian Tribune,* August 10, 2014, p. 1].

Appeal to the Federal Government of Nigeria to close all borders by well meaning groups were not heeded as it was considered draconian. The preventive measures that the different Agencies put in place at the boarders were considered adequate from a public health point of view. What the suggestion revealed was that the management of behaviour change with EVD has to be radically different from the paced pattern of change with the HIV/AIDS epidemic.

Debate over drugs as African medics die of Ebola

The debate over the use of experimental drugs continued as health workers and doctors make up a disproportionate number of those dying of EVD both in the Nigerian outbreak and in the core Ebola outbreak countries of Guinea, Liberia and Sierra Leone [*The Guardian,* August 14, 2014 p. 85]. The death of Sierra Leonean virologist, Dr Sheik Umar Khan, threw the country, and by extension the international community, into a sense of urgency. The impact on the medical and health professions came to the fore when the Nigerian female doctor, Dr. Stella Adadevoh, who had direct contact with index as Senior Consultant at the First Consultant Medical Centre, Ikoyi died of Ebola on Tuesday August 19, 2014 [*The Guardian,* August 20, 2014 p, 1].

Ironically, a day before the death of Dr. Adadevoh occurred, the control of the spread of the Ebola virus appeared to have turned the corner with the announcement that "4 more patients survive Ebola – had been discharged from Lagos quarantine centre, making a total of 5 who had survived; including 2 male doctors and one female nurse who participated in the treatment of Patient Zero [*The Guardian,* August 19, 2014 p. 1]. Nigerian response to experimental drugs

On the day that the US Ambassador to Nigeria, James F. Entwistle, announced at a press briefing that there was not enough trial drug for Nigeria, he added that the Lagos State and Federal governments' responses were just the right one "the isolation ward, screening and especially important that now your government is doing a very good job on this contact tracing." The drug he was referring to is the "ZMapp, being developed by Mapp Biopharmaceutical Inc., It is an experimental treatment for use with individuals infected with Ebola virus. It has not yet been tested in humans for safety or effectiveness. The product, according to the US Centre for Disease Control and Prevention, is a combination of three different monoclonal antibodies that bind to the protein of the Ebola virus" [*The Guardian,* August 19, 2014, p.2].

In response to the emerging drug situation, the Federal government was reported to have deployed the Japanese treatment which most people were hearing about for the first time. The Japanese drug according to a member of the National Committee on Ebola (Professor Maurice Iwu) had passed phase two clinical trials and has been accepted by the Committee for use in treating patients in the country. The same member reported that he had been working on bitter kola nut and would reactivate the project with or without government support. He added that it was wrong to call bitter kola or any other medication a cure at that point. In 1999, prior to the current West African outbreak, his laboratory had found that a component of Garcinia kola called kolaviron was able to inhibit the growth of Ebola. The product is Garcinia IHP [*The Guardian*, August 19, 2014, p.2].

Similarities and differences between the HIV/AIDS epidemic and the EVD outbreak

To appreciate the urgency and stringent control measures that were increasingly being advocated and their borderline ethical justification, attention should be paid to some of the features of the EVD which distinguishes it from the HIV/AIDS. It is on the basis of the differences that forced control of behaviour is based rather than informed behaviour change advocated in the 4-stage framework and on which the central thesis of this book is based. However, there is room for the application of the 4-stage framework to the management of behaviour change in spite of those differences.

In common with the HIV, Ebola Virus (EV) was introduced into the human population from animal reservoirs. According to the WHO, EV is introduced into the human population through close contact with the blood, secretion, organs or other bodily fluids of infected animals. In Africa, infection has been documented through handling of infected chimpanzees, gorillas, fruit bats, monkeys, forest antelope and porcupines found ill or dead in the rain forest.

It is spread in the human community through human to human transmission with infection resulting from direct contact (through broken skin or mucous membranes) with the blood, secretion, organs or other bodily fluids of infected people and indirect contact with environments contaminated with such fluids.

Burial ceremonies in which mourners have direct contact with the body of the deceased person can also play a role in the transmission of Ebola virus. This is a feature which has not been demonstrated for HIV/AIDS.

Incubation period

Although the Ebola virus has a short incubation period in the human before it kills most of the hosts, outside the human body, the viability of the virus is estimated at between five to six hours [former Head of CDC in a CNN interview on October 6, 2014]. Once in the human system, there is generally no detectable symptom for two to three days. This short timeline contrasts sharply with the period of up to six months before HIV can be detected in the human host.

The first symptoms easily detectable but with no assurance of infection is a spike increase in body temperature. Other symptoms such as vomiting, diarrhoea, rashes and unusual bleeding mark the advanced stages of EVD. Death is likely to occur within 21 days of infection. This is another feature which marks EVD apart from HIV/AIDS and carries enormous implications for the notion of orderly and stage change of behaviour. The short timeline and the high fatality of EVD produce the clustering of deaths as a result of the short life cycle of EVD. This compels the use of external forces to put constraint on individual behaviour so as to break the chain of infection. Because of the protracted and variable time line from HIV infection to eventual death, there is no comparable clustering of deaths except in very high HIV prevalence populations. This clustering of deaths creates a panic situation which requires some forceful control to manage. The panic however can be minimized and managed successfully if the public health system takes proactive measures before the arrival of an outbreak.

Pathways/Progression

In much the same pathway as the HIV, Ebola infection depletes the body's immune cells in particular CD4 and CD8 T lymphocytes, which are crucial to the functioning of the immune system.

Protocol for Treatment of EVD patients

The standard WHO protocol for the treatment of EVD patients includes barrier medicine and barrier nursing, fluid and electrolyte replacement, and improving nutrition and micronutrient supplementation [*The Guardian,* August 20, 2014, p. 2]. The problem, however, is that barrier medicine and nursing go against the basic feature of health caring with which health workers are familiar by training and by human intuition.

Fatality rate over time

According to WHO updates since the beginning of the West Africa outbreak, the fatality rates have varied between 60 and 90 percent of those infected. Fatality impacts on panic and prioritization of the EVD.

In short the main difference between the EVD outbreak and the HIV/AIDS epidemic is the extremely short time frame within which EVD consumes a target population or burns out if the chain of transmission from person to person is not broken.

With reference to those who have been cured of Ebola, the WHO indicated that men who have recovered from the disease can still transmit the virus through their semen for up to seven weeks after recovery [*Nigerian Tribune*, August 10, 2014, p. 12]. But the CDC says the virus can still be found in male survivors up to 101 days after the onset of symptoms (m.ibtimes.com/can ebola-spread-through-semen?).

The links between the West African and Nigerian outbreaks

One synergy between the West African and the Nigerian outbreaks was the grim projection of the former which was already in its fourth month having started in March 2014. By the months of August and September, the discovery of new cases in the three mature outbreaks was assumed to be applicable to the Nigerian situation. Table 10.1 shows the dynamics of the outbreak in those countries with widespread transmission.

Table 10.1: Case counts of countries with widespread transmission as of October 29, 2014 (Updated October 31, 2014

Country	Total Cases	Laboratory-Confirmed Cases	Total Deaths
Guinea	1,667*	1,409	1,018
Liberia	6,535	2,515	2,413
Sierra Leone	5,338	3,778	1,510
Total	13,540*	7,702	4,941

Source: *http://www.cdc.gov/vhf/ebola/outbreaks/2014-west-africa/case-counts.html*

Case counts updated in conjunction with the World Health Organisation updates and are based on information reported by the Ministries of Health.

Twenty five days after the arrival of PS in the country and the tracking of primary and secondary contacts of PS, government confirmed 198 Ebola contacts – 177 in Lagos, 21 in Enugu [*The Guardian*, August 14, 2014, pp. 1-2]. A related development was the sense of urgency bordering on panic with which various groups assessed their situation with regards to the tracking exercise and the preparedness of various states to the challenges which have been demonstrated to be enormous but surmountable by the Lagos and Federal MOH collaboration in the Ebola response. The Governor of Lagos met with diplomats, monarchs, others, seeking their views on how to prevent the spread of the outbreak [*The Guardian*, August 14, 2014, p, 83].

At the West African regional level, the issue of closing borders received some attention. On August 19, 2014, the BBC News Channel reported that Cameroun closed her border with Nigeria. The WHO in repeated updates recommended that closing boarders would be counterproductive as resources for tackling the outbreak needed to flow into the affected countries.

The most interesting events of the week were various predictions of impending doom in Nigeria as a result of the index case from Liberia. Ken Isaacs, the spokesman of Samaritan's Purse warned the US Congress that "Ebola is going to emerge with a fury in Nigeria in about three weeks (i.e. early September) due to Sawyer's case" (*The Guardian*, August, 19, 2014, p. 59). The US CDC also issued a Level 2 Travel Alert on Nigeria, warning travellers to take precautionary measures to minimize their risks of contracting the disease.

Ironically, by the end of August, the Ebola Virus Outbreak was nearly under control with a total of 21 cases and 7 deaths according to the WHO update of September 4 covering cases as at August 31, 2014. And on September 30 on the very day the US CDC acknowledged the first EVD case in US, the Federal Ministry of Health announced that the EVD outbreak had been brought under control with no new cases since August 30, 2014.

As further proof, the situation was to be monitored for another 21 days. The WHO confirmed the conclusion reached and on October 20, 2014 declared that Nigeria was Ebola free. The US CDC was so impressed that it sent a team to Nigeria to study the contact tracking system put in place by the Lagos and Federal Health and allied agencies in collaboration with the Partner international agencies.
Contact tracing as the magic bullet

Below are some of the international reactions to the feat of bringing the Nigerian outbreak to an end:

> According to the CDC Director, Tom Frieden "[B]ecause of a rapid public health response, effectively tracking nearly 900 contacts, it appears they have] been able to stop the outbreak in Nigeria," "Though we can't give the all clear yet, it does look like the outbreak is over there. I'm confident that wherever we apply the fundamental principles of infection control in public health, we can stop Ebola."

Nigeria's success appears to be rooted in "contact tracing" – determining every single person that Patrick Sawyer, or Patient Zero, had contact with, and then monitoring them for signs of the virus.

> *"Contact tracing can stop the Ebola outbreak in its tracks," a chart distributed by the CDC declares."*

> *Now contact tracers are at work in the US, setting out to track down as many as 100 people who may have been exposed to Thomas Duncan, who traveled from Liberia to Dallas, where he was eventually diagnosed with the virus (The New York Times)*

> It is an immense task. *The Washington Post* outlines how it went in Nigeria:

> From that single patient came a list of 281 people, [Gavin MacGregor-Skinner, who helped with the Ebola response in Nigeria]. Every one of those individuals had to provide health authorities twice-a-day updates about their well-being, often through methods like text-messaging. Anyone who didn't feel well or failed to respond was checked on, either through a neighborhood network or health workers.

"...In the end, contact tracers – trained professionals and volunteers – conducted 18,500 face-to-face visits to assess potential symptoms, according to the CDC, and the list of contacts throughout the country grew to 894. Two months later, Nigeria ended up with a total of 20 confirmed or probable cases and eight deaths" (*Christian Science Monitor,* October 6, 2014 1:49 pm).

The Nigerian experience was truly remarkable because at about a month after arrival of PS in the country a junior medical officer was discharged on August 18, 2014 after being cleared of infection and was reported to be fine by colleagues *(The Guardian,* August 18, 2014, pp. 1, 4). The next day witnessed 4 more confirmed patients of Ebola discharged by the Federal Minister of Health including two doctors, one nurse who treated Sawyer and a female patient in the hospital at the time the index was on admission, making five such patients who had been cleared of their EV infection within 30 days of the arrival of PS *(Nigerian Tribune,* August 19, 2014, p.3).

In response to the imperfect understanding of the public about just what was involved in the quarantine of suspects in isolation centres and the mounting complaints about features of the medical response, the Governor of Lagos State made a TV appearance during which he addressed the various complaints. The text of the broadcast was published and formed the basis of the following aspects of the broadcast:

Title: For the Record: Our efforts to manage Ebola crisis

- A series of allegations – victims being neglected, useful vaccine or drug being rejected or that there is a shortage of funds – were being made and according to the governor, "None of these is true."
- Ebola did not break out in Nigeria but was imported.
- All contacts have been followed: "We had to react in a proper and methodical way according to acceptable global health standards."
- The state has received help and advice from technical partners – WHO, MSF, CDC – who have tracked the disease for decades: "Our response is a lot better than when the news first broke and our capacity is increasing daily."
- From August 11, daily meetings have been held with stakeholders in the society – traditional and religious leaders, market men and women etc. – to brief them of the risk and to reassure them that "we are daily gaining control, and to advise all not to panic but (be) cautious."
- The Governor complemented the courage of health workers, their professionalism, patriotism and humanitarian disposition.
- He appreciated the concern of relatives of those under surveillance but pointed out that they were receiving the best care experts had recommended.
- He warned opportunists doing brisk business on the back of the outbreak to desist from such activities.

· He affirmed that there was no fund shortage and that the President and Federal MOH are both aware of national and global risk and have shown appropriate will by providing additional resources if asked.

· He observed that the Nigerian outbreak was the first urban appearance of the disease and an opportunity to show the world how to overcome it.

- *The Guardian,* August 18, 2014, p. 11).

Infection of Western health and aid workers

During the fifth week of the Nigerian outbreak, developments surrounding the infection of foreign health workers in the core EVD zones of Guinea, Sierra Leone and Liberia dominated world attention. Finally, beyond the movement of PS to Nigeria, repatriation of infected people to their home countries revealed the enormity of the resource needs of coping with a potential EVD epidemic. A specially fitted plane was needed to move a single US citizen back home for treatment.

Another side effect of the globalization of the outbreak was to bring the drug politics into sharper relief. Whilst the repatriated patients were allowed use of the ZMapp, supply to meet the needs of the West African outbreak was impracticable because of ethical and logistic issues. US would not authorise its use on ethical grounds and the manufacturers did not have the stock to supply those needs. And the building up of stock of the ZMapp was estimated to take a long time for which the outbreak could not wait.

The international response under the potential threat to the complacency of Europe and the US was to make a more aggressive move to provide some support in human and material support to the worst affected countries. Unfortunately, it is easy to pledge fund but much more problematic to fulfil those pledges. The UK EVD meeting tried to resolve this dilemma and made relatively more progress because of the demonstrable vulnerability of Europe by this time.

Season of good news
Then towards the middle of August, two pieces of news came out, one encouraging the other disturbing. It was reported that antibodies from Ebola survivors could provide effective therapies [*The Guardian,* August 28, 2014, p.1). It was also reported that the personal protective equipment used for barrier nursing may not fully shield health workers from infection (*The Guardian,* August 29, 2014, p.1).

The news was followed by others. Another newspaper reported the cheering news that a Doctor (in desperation and inspiration) treated Ebola patient with HIV drug in Liberia. Lamivudine was given to 15 EVD infected patients and only 2 died giving a mortality rate of 7% compared to the prevailing 70% across West Africa (*Nigerian Tribune,* August 29, 2014, p. 47). And on September 5, 2014, it was reported that WHO expected that as a result of the fast tracking of clinical testing as many as 8 possible treatments and 2 vaccines were now available (*Nigerian Tribune,* September 5, 2014, p 47).

To crown 60 days of roller coaster concern about the Nigerian Ebola outbreak, the Federal Minister of Health on September 23, 2014 seized the occasion of the United Nations General Assembly holding in New York, USA to announce that Nigeria was completely free of active Ebola (EVD) cases, stating further that all contacts of the deadly disease have been released from scrutiny. In the minister's words:

> "Presently, there is no single case of Ebola virus disease in Nigeria – none. No cases are under treatment, no suspected cases. There are no contacts in Lagos that are still under surveillance, having completed a minimum of 21 days of observation.

> "None of them is showing any symptoms. Monday (22 September, 2014) will mark the end of their 21 days of observation and the plan is to get them discharged from surveillance yesterday (Tuesday 23 September 2014). Nigeria will be as clean as any other country as far as Ebola virus disease is concerned." (September 24, 2014 posted by Datboyjerry) Read more at http://www.360nobs.com/2014/09/health-minister-declares-nigeria-ebola-free/#uith6fQTjdr473XT.99)

He added that although Nigeria had been able to successfully contain the virus, preventing stigmatization of Ebola survivors remained a challenge.

On the management of contact tracking so as to obtain the cooperation and compliance of those under observation, he added:

> "Three terms became part of our lexicon: surveillance, quarantine, and isolation. Surveillance is sort of like house arrest. You don't criminalize them. The person is actually a victim, not a criminal. We monitor their movements, the rest of the family are counselled about what contact can and can't be done. We have contact with them every day. You can imagine what this effort must have been like when we had 300 in Lagos and over 400 in Port Harcourt.
> "That is the first time we are denying that individual the comfort of his own bed. We put him in separately from the isolation ward from those who are confirmed. If malaria, we discharge them to their doctor to be treated for malaria," the minister explained (*Ibid.*).

Then on October 20, which marked 42 days since Nigeria's last confirmed Ebola case and at twice the 21-day incubation period, the country was declared free of the EVD that had ravaged three West African neighbours by the WHO (https://uk.news.yahoo.com/why-nigeria-able-beat-ebola-not-boko-haram-182239564--politics.html#0TS464s).

QUESTIONS ARISING

1.   Is it all over?

The first major question arising from the control of the "first" Nigerian EVD outbreak is to ask if the end of new cases implies that the threat of the EVD is over or if there will be subsequent outbreaks even if they are equally efficiently managed. The answer on the basis of common sense will be that if the so called end of the outbreak is taken literarily, complacency in control measures at borders, in personal life and in the preparedness for facing an outbreak will set in. That layman view is backed by the epidemiological imperative that with the ease of movement of persons all over the world, no amount of infrared temperature taking can assure the certainty of preventing entry of persons with the virus as long as the outbreak is still ravaging other countries in the region and elsewhere in the world.

2.   What role did behaviour change play in control of EVD so far?

An associated question more relevant to the behaviour change focus of this book is to go behind the obvious logic of contact tracing and quarantine approach to the control of the EVD. It is worth noting that contact tracing was used in other public health circumstances with limited effectiveness in the past as means of control of those circumstances. A case in point is the attempt to use contact tracing for controlling the spread of STIs. The tool was used much more in the most common place instances of gonorrhoea and less so with the HIV/AIDS epidemic. Why was this so?

The answer can be found in the different images that society and individuals attach to different diseases. In the case of sexually transmitted infections, the common STIs such as gonorrhoea were not fatal and were considered almost as a badge of honour among young people. In contrast HIV/AIDS is considered as more serious and attracted stigma on the basis of the moral judgement attached to the infection.

The other reason is that contact tracing is a sensitive tool in limited spatial scope and becomes less sensitive in widespread dissemination of an outbreak among a rapidly mobile population of the type that occupy border areas and in post war situation such as along the borders of the three most affected countries of Guinea, Sierra Leone and Liberia.

These features of contact tracing bring attention to the issue of using behaviour change as an essential tool of limiting and containing an epidemic or outbreak. The lessons of the control of the Nigerian outbreak and the ongoing struggle to cope with what amounts to a raging epidemic of the disease in the three countries most affected by the outbreak are many. They all touch on the flexibility of human ethics and the psychology of survival when it comes to changing behaviour through persuasion or through the brutal use of force so as to achieve public health objectives.

The flexibility in human ethics spills over into decisions of the type that surrounds the ongoing debate about the use of pre-trial drugs. It was a factor in the innovative use of HIV drug Lamivudine for treating EVD patients. It is also a factor in the fast tracking of clinical testing of candidate treatment and vaccines. As pointed out earlier, such pushing of the ethical envelope is not always disastrous. It can be argued that it is equally ethically right to take these chances because of the urgency of the situation when doing nothing is not an option.

Consequently it may be argued that the virulence of Ebola virus and the short cycle of infection to death leaves very narrow range of options within the fine points of ethics relating to spread of infection, the activities of communities and basic rights of individual versus the common good to be subject to extended or in depth discussion.

On the other hand it may be argued that since knowledge of phenomenon contributes to the development of ethical values around it, there should be no ethical flexibility blamed on the short cycle of the disease life history. The parameters of Ebola virus disease outbreaks have been known since 1976. It took the 2014 West African outbreak to reveal the discriminatory ethical values on which policies and programmes of coping with an outbreak were based. As long as such outbreaks were limited to isolated rural communities where the virus burns itself out, making elaborate drug and vaccine preparedness plans was financially unattractive. This is one of the logical explanations of the limited levels of anticipation in the US and Western Europe that the outbreak could reach their door steps. For future outbreaks or in response to the current outbreak anticipatory plans can be put in place some of which become more ethically sound than has been the case.

Another redeeming feature of the hasty ethical decisions such as those behind WHO approval of drugs or the fast tracking of drug testing and deployment is the extremely high fatality rates that obtain in the absence of a decent health infrastructure that can implement the basic treatment protocol for EVD. The high fatality among health workers also raises the ethical approach to the training of such workers for the common as well as for the uncommon diseases. Obviously the demands for barrier nursing and care were limited prior to the highly contagious Ebola virus outbreak.

Obviously, if there are barriers to arriving at a global value of the common good in social and economic terms, then emergency government action in the name of local common good will pose problems for the sustenance of common good.

In the same way finding a middle ground between any common good and individual rights will always be difficult. The individual rights are often structured in terms of the habits and familiar social values of the individual whereas the attainment of the common good, often requires a drastic rearrangement of those habits and values. This is particularly true of the response to the management of the EVD outbreak: individuals are separated from their family, friends and community; mothers cannot stay with sick children or children go to comfort sick relatives; cremation is substituted for the ritual of sending off the dead with close and loving attention.

It is not going to be easy to relax some of these stringent preventive methods, but with the tools of persuasion within behaviour change, it is possible to be more proactive in preparing the communities for those changes for the sake of management of future outbreaks of any epidemic or outbreak. The bottom line though is that the adequacy of any measures put in place depends on their being tried and tested. Unfortunately, these epidemics and outbreaks are far between although the outbreaks are getting more frequent.

CONCLUSION: How does the 4-Stage Framework align with the needs of the EVD outbreak?

Stage 1: It is now clear that being aware of outbreaks in other countries, and even participating in the management of the outbreaks does not fully prepare individuals, communities or governments for the crucial 4-stage framework stage of establishing vulnerability through self risk assessment. But if there is a deliberate effort to prepare for staged behaviour change, then lessons must be drawn from ongoing outbreaks as inputs into the management of subsequent outbreaks.

Stage 2: Under the fast moving scenario of an Ebola virus outbreak, limited self risk assessment needs to be supplemented by rapid dissemination of change agents side by side with the short term effort to disseminate the necessary information for survival. In effect the second and third stages of the 4-stage framework overlap in the mind of the public. The challenge is to be able to phrase risk in the proper proportion so that factual information does not get exaggerated into scare tactics.

Certainly Ebola virus disease kills. But the circumstances of exposure need to be specified in clear physical and social terms so that people can make informed decisions as to when they are exposed. As in the case of HIV/AIDS, communicating the fine points of viability of virus on stair rails, door knobs and the like requires a new language of passing on scientific facts to lay people.

Fear of death is one of the strongest emotions when people assess the seriousness of any threat and their personal vulnerability. The high fatality associated with Ebola and the horrible physical manifestations in the last phase of the disease leading to death tend to encourage a conservative attitude to taking care in avoiding infection. Consequently, allaying fears of the public is not achieved by false assurances. The more clearly the odds people face are explained, the more likely they will be able to make realistic assessment of their safety in different circumstances.

Stage 3: The dissemination of information on features of the EVD, the services which are available for the prevention of infection and the facilities for testing for infection and gaining admission into the quarantine units constitute a large body of knowledge.

The challenge is the short period of time available for achieving saturation at all levels of society and at relevant points of service. The segmentation of the audience by literacy, urban and rural residence and by predisposing cultural practices are some of the problems that have to be coped with within the short period available for assuring familiarity with procedures.

The inefficiencies in information dissemination is partly responsible for the enforcement of the final Stage 4 in which the behaviour change takes place not on the basis of informed consent but on the basis of the logic and priorities of the dangers posed by the epidemic. However, these enforced behaviour changes can be made more palatable if people are given competent and informed counselling by those responsible for processing them through the preventive and curative systems. These counselling skills are also required by the staff handling borders and by law enforcement agencies. Such skills should be built into the training of health and other workers required for the management of epidemics and outbreaks prior to their arrival.

Stage 4: As a result of the compression of events in an outbreak such as the EVD, the final stage of behaviour change of the type advocated in this book is a shared responsibility between individuals, the common good and the government. The threat from the outbreak was severe enough to break down the resistance of the individuals to the restrictions and reduction of their rights. However, a residual resentment remains because the enforced behaviour change is not voluntary. This feature explains why those who are infected, including people with medical and health education still find ways of compromising the restricting system put in place.

The implication of these modifications to the persuasive behaviour change is that processes should be in place with which to cope with outbreaks as part of the health system readiness and not as panic reaction to the arrival of an outbreak. It is pertinent to mention that Nigeria may not have seen the last of the West African outbreak, but the systems with which she controlled the this particular outbreak are actively being studied by other countries and should be preserved by Nigeria in readiness for that possible repeat.

One beauty of the 4-stage framework is that it exposes the gaps in preparedness for outbreaks even in the advanced countries with supposedly advanced health systems. Otherwise, it is difficult to appreciate why the UK had only one Unit in North London which was ready to cope with EVD patients. It also explains why the uneven preparedness for handling EVD cases in the US is becoming an embarrassment. Both the US and the UK certainly did not get the vulnerability from EVD outbreak right. In contrast the WHO list of African countries which are prepared for EVD is a reflection of the national vulnerability assessment that such countries have made. The list includes the east African travel hubs of Kenya and Ethiopia.

A loophole apparently exists in the reliance on barrier nursing and care in the observation, testing and caring for suspected or infected persons. This is likely explanation of the transmission of infection in Madrid, Spain and on US soil from Duncan to a nurse in similar circumstances (BBC TV, Sunday, October 12, 2014). It has been suggested that the kits may not be perfect, or that the protocol for putting on and taking off the kit may be unknowingly breached due to possible flaws in the training of staff. In Spain the nurse was suspected to have touched her face with the infected glove when she was taking off the head piece. These mishaps suggests that the health workers require workplace behaviour change as much as the general population need to change some habits so as to cope with emerging challenges of health hazards in the community.

CONCLUSION

It is hoped that the Part 1 of the book demonstrated the soundness of the theoretical underpinnings of the 4-stage framework and that the performance of the model on various projects detailed in chapters 6 to 10 proved the robustness of its application in different settings. The advent of the Nigeria EVD outbreak created an exception and a novel situation in which the time for orderly change of behaviour was not long enough nor did the natural history of the disease allow such voluntary personal responses.

However, this final chapter attempted to fit the outbreak albeit imperfectly into the 4-Stage framework with the caution that anticipating outbreaks and building coping scenarios for them is the way to achieve a compromise between the stringency of conditions for managing the outbreak and creating the environment in which people will understand the restriction on their rights but be willing to cooperate for their self preservation even if not for the common good.

It is quite possible to think of other health situations in which the 4-stage framework might be a valid framework for sustained behaviour change needed to achieve given health outcomes. Some of the sexual and reproductive health outcomes require substantial behaviour change that has proved resistant to the prevailing behaviour changing communication strategies of the types reviewed in Part 1 of the book. The 4-stage framework can inform the restructuring of behaviour change in such aspects as antenatal and post natal care and even in child care so that the goals of improved outcomes can be within reach.

Table 10.2: Latest figures of the world wide foot print of EVD – Euronews TV 10-10-14)

COUNTRY	CASES	DEATHS	FATALITY RATES (%)
WEST AFRICAN OUTBREAK			
Liberia	3924-	2316	59.0
Sierra Leone	2789-	930	33.3
Guinea	1298	778	59.9
Democratic Republic Of Congo	71	43	60.5
Nigeria	20	8	40.0
Senegal	1	0	0.0
OUTSIDE WEST AFRICA			
Spain	3	2	66.6
France	1	0	0.0
Norway	1	0	0.0
Germany	1	0	0.0
United Kingdom	1	0	0.0
United States	4	1	25.0

Source: Euronews TV, October 10, 2014.

REFERENCES

Adedimeji, A T., Jagha, E. Weiss, L. Adeokun and J. Mantell, (2001). "Perceptions of HIV/AIDS risks among Family Planning Clients in Ibadan, Nigeria." Abstract accepted at the IUSSP Conference, July 24-26, Salvador, Brazil.

Adeokun, Lawrence. A. (1982). "Marital sexual relationships and birth spacing among two Yoruba sub-groups, Africa." *Journal of the International Institute of African Languages and Cultures,* January 1, 1982.

Adeokun, Lawrence A. *(2009). Sociocultural Aspects of Family Planning and HIV/ AIDS in Nigeria.* ABBI Books, Ibadan, Nigeria, 2009.

Adeokun Lawrence, Joanne E. Mantell, Eugene Weiss, Grace Ebun Delano, Temple Jagha, Jumoke Olatoregun, Dora Udo, Stella Akinso and Ellen Weiss (2002). "Promoting Dual Protection in Family Planning Clinics in Ibadan, Nigeria." *International Family Planning Perspectives*, Volume 28, Number 2, June, 2002 (Issues in Perspective).

Agbaje J. B. (2005). "The Place of Yorùbá Proverbs in the Understanding of Yorùbá Philosophy and Education." *International Journal of African and African American Studies,* 1 (5): 48-54.

Ajzen, I. and M. Fishbein (1980). *Understanding attitudes and predicting social behavior.* Englewood Cliffs, NJ: Prentice-Hall.

Bandura, Albert *(1982).* "Self-efficacy Mechanism in Human Agency." *American Psychologist* 37:122-47.

Bandura, A. (1988). "Organisational applications of social cognitive theory." *Australian Journal of Management, 13,* 275-302.

Bandura, A. (1988). "Perceived self-efficacy: Exercise of control through self-belief." In J. P. Dauwalder, M. Perrez, and V. Hobi (Eds.), *Annual series of European research in behavior therapy* (Vol. 2, pp. 27-59). Amsterdam/Lisse, Netherlands: Swets & Zeitlinger.

Bankole, Naomi (1982). "Conceptual problems in nutrition education in Western Nigeria." *Food Policy,* vol. 7, issue 4, pp. 323-331.

Bounds, W., J. Guillebaud, L. Stewart, et al. (1988). "A female condom (Femshield): A study of its user acceptability." *British Journal of Family Planning 14:83– 87.*

Bounds, W. (1989). "Male and Female Condoms." *British Journal of Family Planning,* 15:14-17.

Bulatao R. A. (1998). The Value of Family Planning Programs in Developing Countries. Santa Monica, CA: RAND.

Caldwell, John C., Pat Caldwell and I. O. Orubuloye (1992). "The Family and Sexual Networking in Sub-Saharan Africa: Historical Regional Differences and Present-Day Implications." *Population Studies,* 46 no. 3: 385-410.

Cates W and K. M. Stone (1992). "Family planning, sexually transmitted diseases and contraceptive choice: A literature update – part I." *Fam Plann Perspect* 1992; 24(2):75- 84.

Cates W. (1996). "Contraception, unintended pregnancy and sexually transmitted diseases: Why isn't a simple solution possible?" *Am J Epidemiology,* 1996; 143(4):311- 18.

Cates W. (1996). "Contraceptive choice, sexually transmitted diseases, HIV infection and future fecundity." *JBr Fertil Soc* 1996; 1(1):18-22.

Center for Disease Control and Prevention (2010). "Ebola Hemorrhagic Fever Fact Sheet." Available at: http://www.cdc.gov/ncidod/dvrd/spb/mnpages/dispages/Fact_Sheets/ Ebola_Fact_Booklet.pdf

Christian Science Monitor (2014*).* "Nigeria contains Ebola – and US officials want to know more." By Ariel Zirulnick, October 6, 2014 1:49 PM.

Cichocki. "The History of Condoms: Centuries of Safer Sex" (http://aids.about.com/od/ condominformation/qt/condomhistory.htm).

Ehrhardt, A. A. and T. M. Exner (2000). "Prevention of sexual risk behavior for HIV infection with women." *AIDS,* 14(Suppl.), S53-S58.

Essien E. James, Angela F. Meshack, Ronald J. Peters, G. O. Ogungbade and Nora I. Osemene (2005). "Strategies to prevent HIV transmission among heterosexual African-American women." *International Journal for Equity in Health,* 2005, 4:4, p. 28.

Farr, G., H. Gabelnick, K. Sturgen and L. Dorflinger (1994). "Contraceptive efficacy and acceptability of the female condom." *American Journal of Public Health,* 84, 1960–1964.

Federal Ministry of Health, Nigeria (1991). National HIV Seroprevalence Sentinel Survey. Abuja: Federal Ministry of Health.

Federal Ministry of Health, Nigeria (1999). National HIV Seroprevalence Sentinel Survey. Abuja: Federal Ministry of Health.

Federal Ministry of Health, Nigeria (2001). National HIV Seroprevalence Sentinel Survey. Abuja: Federal Ministry of Health.

Federal Ministry of Health, Nigeria (2003). National HIV Seroprevalence Sentinel Survey. Abuja: Federal Ministry of Health.

Federal Ministry of Health, Nigeria (2005). Technical Report on the 2003 National HIV Seroprevalence Sentinel Survey. Abuja: Federal Ministry of Health.

Federal Ministry of Health, Nigeria (2008). National HIV Seroprevalence Sentinel Survey, Abuja: Federal Ministry of Health.

Federal Ministry of Health, Nigeria (2010). National HIV Sentinel Survey Among Pregnant Women. Abuja: Federal Ministry of Health.

Federal Ministry of Health (2012) National HIV & AIDS and Reproductive Health Survey (NARHS Plus II). Abuja: Federal Ministry of Health.

FHI (2003). "Examining the Influence of Providers on Contraceptive Uptake in Rwanda." November, 2013.

Fishbein, M. and I. Ajzen (1975). *Belief, attitude, intention, and behavior: An introduction to theory and research.* Reading, MA: Addison-Wesley.

Fitch, J.T. (2001). "Are Condoms Effective in Reducing the Risk of Sexually Transmitted Disease?" *The Annals of Pharmacotherapy,* September 2001, Volume 35:1136-8.

Gerrard, M., F. X. Gibbons, and B. J. Bushman (1996). "Relation between perceived vulnerability to HIV and precautionary sexual behavior." *Psychological Bulletin, 119,* 390-409.

Gordon, Christopher M., Michael P. Carey and Kate B. Carey (1997). "Effects of a drinking event on behavioral skills and condom attitudes in men: Implications for HIV risk from a controlled experiment." *Health Psychology,* Vol 16(5), Sept 1997, 490-495.

Graeff, Judith Allen, John P. Elder, Elizabeth Mills Booth (1993). *Health Communication (Program)* Jossey-Bass Publishers, 1993 - *Health & Fitness* - 204 pages.

Hoffman, Sarah Z. (2004). "HIV/AIDS in Cuba: a model for care or an ethical dilemma?" *Afr Health Sci.* Dec., 2004; 4(3): 208-209.

Jagha, T; J. Mantell, L. Adeokun, E. Weiss, A. Adedimeji (2001). "STI/HIV/AIDS Knowledge, Risk Perception and Condom Use among Family Planning Clinics in Osogbo, Nigeria." Abstract accepted at the 8th AIDS IMPACT Conference, July 8-11, 2001, Brighton, UK.

Kebaabetswe, P. and Noor, Kathleen F. (2002). "Behavioral Change: Goals and Means." Chapter 33 in *AIDS in Africa* (Second Edition) by Max Essex *et. al.* (eds). Kluwer Academic/Plenum Publishers, New York.

Kippax S., J. Noble, G. Prestage, J. M. Crawford, D. Campbell, D. Baxter and D. Cooper (1997). "Sexual negotiation in the AIDS era: negotiated safety revisited." AIDS. Feb. 1997, 11(2):191-7.

Lewin, K. (1935). *A dynamic theory of personality.* New York: McGraw-Hill. Lewin, K. (1936). *Principles of topological psychology.* New York: McGraw-Hill.

Lewin, K. and R. Lippitt (1938). "An experimental approach to the study of autocracy and democracy: A preliminary note," *Sociometry* 1: 292-300.

Lewin, K., R. Lippitt and R. White (1939). "Patterns of aggressive behaviour in experimentally created social climates,'" *Journal of Social Psychology,* 10: 271-99.

Lewin, K. and Grabbe, P. (*1945*). "Conduct, knowledge, and acceptance of new values," *Journal of Social Issues,* 1, 3, pp. 53-64.

Lewin, K. (1947). "Frontiers of Group Dynamics: Concept, method and reality in social science, social equilibria, and social change." *Human Relations,* 1, 5-41.

Lewin, I. (1948). *Resolving social conflicts; selected papers on group dynamics.* In Gertrude W. Lewin (ed.). New York: Harper& Row, 1948.

Lewin, K. (1951). *Field theory in social science; selected theoretical papers.* D. Cartwright (Ed.). New York: Harper& Row.

Mantell, J., E. Weiss, L. Adeokun, G. Delano, T. Jagha, Olatoregun, G. Ishola, (2000). "Dual protection in Family Planning Clinics: Operations Research from Nigeria." Poster presentations at the 13th International AIDS Conference, Durban, South Africa, 9-14, July 2000.

Mantell, J., E. Weiss, L. Adeokun, G. Delano, D. Udo, S. Akinso (2000). "Introducing the female condom within family planning clinics in Nigeria." Poster presentations at the 13th International AIDS Conference, Durban, South Africa, 9-14, July 2000.

Mantell, J., E. Weiss, L. Adeokun, G. Delano, T. Jagha (2000). "Evaluating the feasibility of promoting dual protection practices in Nigeria." Poster presentations at the 13th International AIDS Conference Durban, South Africa, 9-14, July 2000.

Mantell, J., E. Weiss, L. Adeokun, G. Delano, T. Jagha, Olatoregun., G. Ishola, and K. Akinpelu (2001). "The impact of male gender roles on HIV risks in South West Nigeria." Paper presented at the annual meeting of the American Public Health Association, Atlanta, GA, USA, Oct. 21-25, 2001.

Mantell Joanne E., Shari L. Dworkin, Theresa M. Exner, Susie Hoffman, Jenni A. Smit, and Ida Susser (2006). "The promises and limitations of female-initiated methods of HIV/STI protection." *Social Science and Medicine.* Oct 2006; 63(8): 1998–2009.

Meekers D. and M. Oladosu (1996). "Spousal communication and family planning decision-making in Nigeria." University Park, Pennsylvania, Pennsylvania State University,

Population Research Institute, 1996 Apr 15. [3], 33 (Population Research Institute Working Papers in African Demography, Working Paper AD96-03).

Messersmith L. J., T. T. Kane, A. I. Odebiyi and A. A. Adewuyi (2000). "Who's at risk? Men's STD experience and condom use in southwest Nigeria." *Stud Fam Plann.* Sep. 2000; 31 (3):203–16.

Microsoft® Encarta® (2009).

Mike Earl-Taylor (2002). "HIV/AIDS, the stats, the virgin cure and infant rape." *Science in Africa,* Africa's First On-Line Science Magazine, MERCK.

Miller, K. S., B. A. Kotchick, S. Dorsey, R. Forehand and A. Y. Ham (1998). "Family communication about sex: What are parents saying and are their adolescents listening?" *Family Planning Perspectives,* 30, 218–222, 235.

Ngo, Leo Babauta. "7 little habits that can change your life and how to form them." Available at: [http://zenhabits.net/7-little-habits-that-can-change-your-life-and-how-to-form-them/]

NIH/CDC Consensus Panel in 2000 Workshop Summary: Scientific Evidence on Condom Effectiveness for Sexually Transmitted Disease (STD) Prevention, June 12-13, 2000, Hyatt Dulles Airport Herndon, Virginia This summary report was prepared by the National Institute of Allergy and Infectious Diseases, National Institute of Health, Department of Health and Human Services. July 20, 2001.

Nwadigwe Charles Emeka (2012). "Theatre for Development: An Alternative Programme for Reproductive Health Communication in Urban Nigeria." *African Sociological Review* 16(2), pp.102-118.

Odutolu, Oluwole (2005). "Convergence of behaviour change models for AIDS risk reduction in sub-Saharan Africa." *Int J Health Plann* Mgmt. 20: 239–252. Published online in Wiley InterScience(www.interscience.wiley.com).

Oladipo, O. (2002). "Public Health Education." In *Health Education and Health Promotion.* Edited by Ademuwagun Z. A. *et. al.* Ibadan Sterling-Horden Publishers (Nig)Ltd.

Papasratorn Borworn. (borworn@computer.org) (2012) "Effect of Age, Culture, and Language on Adoption and Quality of Services of IP based Communication." The First

International Conference on Mobility for Life: Problem Based Learning, Technology and Telecommunications (TT-PBL'11), Chiang Rai, Thailand 5-7 March, 2012.

Prochaska, J.O., C. C. DiClemente and J.C. Norcross (1992). "In search of how people change - applications to addictive behaviors." American Psychologist, 47(9), 1102-1114.

Richey, Lisa Ann (2008). "Global knowledge/local bodies: Family planning service providers' interpretations of contraceptive knowledge(s)." Demographic Research, Volume 18, Article 17, pages 469-498 - Published 10 June, 2008 at: http://www.demographic-research.org/Volumes/Vol18/17/

Rosenstock I., V. Strecher, and M. Becker (1994). "The Health Belief Model and HIV risk behaviour change." In R. J. DiClemente and J. L. Peterson (Eds.), *Preventing AIDS: Theories and methods of behavioural interventions.* New York: Plenum Press, pp. 5-24.

Ross, H.S. & P. R. Mico (1980). *Theory and Practice in Health education,* Palo Alto, California: Mayfield.

Sa Wahid (2006). "How Habits are Formed by Our Mind." Ezine Articles at: http://ezinearticles.com/?How-Habits-are-Formed-by-Our-Mind&id=339888)

Sangi-Haghpeykar H, Horth F, and A. N. Poindexter (2001). "Condom use among sterilized and nonsterilized Hispanic women." *Sex Transm Dis. Sep.,2001, 28(9):546- 51.*

Strobe W. & M. Hewstone (Eds.), *European review of social psychology*, vol 4.

Trussell, J. (1998). "Contraceptive efficacy of the Reality® *female condom. "* *Contraception,* 58:147,*1998.*

INDEX

www.ingramcontent.com/pod-product-compliance
Lightning Source LLC
Chambersburg PA
CBHW080616190526
45169CB00009B/3204